Devoured Soul

Myra A. Jackson

iUniverse, Inc.
New York   Bloomington

iUniverse books may be ordered through booksellers or by contacting:

iUniverse
1663 Liberty Drive
Bloomington, IN 47403
www.iuniverse.com
1-800-Authors (1-800-288-4677)

ISBN: 978-0-595-53154-7 (sc)
ISBN: 978-1-4401-1329-1 (hc)
ISBN: 978-0-595-63216-9 (ebook)

Printed in the United States of America

iUniverse rev. date: 04/17/2009

Contents

Chapter 1
Lack Of Knowledge

"The Failure To Recognize"

Madison's thoughts were so overwhelming it had gotten to the point where lying was the best way to escape the madness. She was so desperate to run for cover; she thought by telling her boss, Vernon she was quitting her job due to family issues would make controlling her emotions easier. That story wasn't the truth. She just didn't have the courage to reveal her pain to those who knowingly allowed personal attacks and harassment to take place between two employees for amusement. Never considering the repercussions it would have on them, and their families. Madison's story begins during the fall of 2001' where she had been dealing with a difficult situation at home with a family member Jesse Walters who was at the time her man and the father of her children. Madison was never one to discuss her personal problems with the neighbors, or strangers feeling it was no others business, but her own. However, she was struggling with a stressful environment at home that inevitably made it impossible to separate the two worlds from colliding. What was about to happen

1

to her next she couldn't begin to comprehend? While unable to remember every clash she had with a woman name Ms. Karen Filcher, 'she was able to remember the fight that brought her where she is today. Hired a few years behind Madison, Karen came to assist in production. Madison didn't know the woman at all or where she had come from she was just introduced to Karen. For Madison she was like any other hire; you train them, show them the ropes and give them space to do their job. What Mattie didn't recall was being told that Karen was already working for the company, or the reason for the position change. What she does remember is being kept in the dark regarding the details of why she was moved to her area. A witty woman who had the ability to be kind and comical in her demeanor was all of a sudden working in QA". Madison didn't mind' hell she needed the help. As the weeks flew by, she would get visits from some of the other co-workers; workers that hardly graced her department before Karen came to work there. In the back of Mattie's mind: She wondered what the attraction was all of sudden, noticing her newfound fan base. However, it didn't take her long to find out. Karen was different she could make you laugh, empathize, and feel sorry for her at one time. But' what Madison saw was a changing soul acting and behaving so, bizarre Madison, became concerned. Something is wrong; Mattie couldn't put her finger on what the problem was. All she knew... was that Karen was different . Madison continued to do her job as she would any other day ignoring the personality conflicts. We continued to work our jobs as usual, but it never went without a glitch. Karen was always energetic, and all over the place, her aggressiveness was even scary at times. The woman's personality changed with the wind so often it was worth paying attention to, because along with that change "came hostility, and anger presumably for not being treated well or something of that nature. Madison heard her complaints of dissatisfaction regarding her personal life, and mistreatment at home regularly shouting and ranting recklessly about being ignored. Mattie couldn't help hearing the anger coming from her. What she had gotten to know about the woman observing her behavior was shocking especially when she expressed it aloud for all to see. Karen's antics were amazing; this woman's sexual connotations... floored Mattie, and some of the workers. Madison thought she was open when it came to expressing herself, but Karen on the other hand was very detailed regarding her taste in men. This wasn't her only topic of conversation she spoke of being less than human' being unwanted, and how family hated the sight of her. The emotional outburst went on for years. Madison was tired of listening to her talking about her boyfriends desires in the bedroom. Karen felt he was hiding something about himself. She put on a show that the average woman wouldn't touch on their worst day; not without shame or embarrassment. Karen seemed to be reaching out any way she could for help. Asking in the only way she knew how, they saw nothing wrong with that. Karen worked hard for that acknowledgement in whatever she did, and getting into trouble was no exception to prove her worthiness to the company. Madison could appreciate when a person went the extra mile on a task and of course, a pat on the back at some point was cool. With this in mind, Mattie was unable to figure out where their acceptance of Kerens behavior became tolerable. She could only guess at what it might be. Madison was in charge of the area, they both did their parts keeping production moving. Karen didn't feel acknowledged adequately for the work she was doing. What she felt was put- off, by their avoidance of her. That avoidance started something for her, and she most definitely wanted Madison to know how she felt about being in her shadow all the time. The assumption is 'Karen is more efficient and skilled to have the position Madison held... this was her argument for causing problems. The downside to that argument was she had no social skill at all, and he wasn't Madison. Karen had no attention span, no discipline to her mouth and she drank like a fish. This observation of Karen's personality issues lead Mattie to believe the woman had been placed with her on purpose to avoid any complications with the last co-worker, which further told her they were dodging a responsibility, and Mattie's suspicions were true; that something was wrong with her. To validate her point of rage, and anger you would have to experience several betrayals as she had. The last few years of contact with Karen, who she gave her time and effort in supporting for reasons she felt were legitimate at the time slowly opened her eyes to see how manipulation, betrayal and denial could change you forever. Madison concluded by acknowledging Karen needed a shoulder to cry on, and she hesitantly allowed Karen to confide in her, because she seemed desperate, however, Madison never agreed to be committed to her need for support forever, just an ear every now and again. After becoming a little more acquainted with Karen, her heartbreaks, and the personal conflicts with family the relationship seemed workable for the two women' …you'd never think there were animosity lurking about. Madison informed Karen, that her family relationship was tight knit… that they had fights, disagreements like anyone else, but they stayed close no matter what. Madison had no problem with sharing, she just felt that her personal life was hers and no others. Going to the job everyday brought a satisfaction to Madison's life, as she stayed sharp, and on top of her day as always. However, for her co-worker that was another story. Time passed, and Karen appeared to be unfocused on some days, or a little tilted which didn't help her problems. The atmosphere was constantly on hiatus with her, because she couldn't get herself together. Madison was consoling sometimes, but wanted to be alone. Karen hated being ignored and voiced this to Madison all the time by shouting her dislike for the avoidance. Karen had become annoying and very rude on purpose for a laugh she bragged all the time of having more experience than Madison, and should have her job. Mattie tuned her out, because she was taking her kindness for granted, and didn't appreciate the disrespect she was shown. Karen needed help, but it wasn't her job to decipher what that was to be. The battle with Karen became more intense as the days passed. The woman had serious issues to the point that no other person wanted to come near her for fear of confrontations. Madison became the problem for Karen, because she refused to walk on eggshells to make her ass happy. The woman had become unruly, and belligerent towards Mattie, and all who crossed her path. This is what Madison had to deal with at least once a week if she were lucky, and most times all week long. As she said, Madison had been working there far longer than Karen without one complaint had. As lead worker Madison had garnered a good repose with management although, she had some attendance issues she needed to handle everything else was good. Management kept her up to date on expectations for the week's shipment and pick-up so they would have it completed early. This is where the problem comes in. Madison's job was to research and verify information through channels along with some labor work. Karen was to audit and report by paper. The work arrangement didn't suite Karen at all. Instead, she wanted Madison's job. Mattie saw through the big performances she gave. Karen loved to amuse the masses with her filthy mouth it was hilarious at times, but she knew what she was doing. The hostility and aggressive behavior had become a common practice she figured it would get her what she wanted; control. Karen lashed out every way she could calling Mattie all the bitches, and dummies she could cram in to her vocabulary to name a few during that time. The storm brewing inside Madison had been simmering for a very long time, due to the lack of support from management. This anger towards management was caused partly by their ineffectiveness to handle Karen's tirades. This deliberate avoidance for the apparent situation furthered Mattie's inability to turn a blind side to the insults flying at her By avoiding Karen , along with the name-calling and taunting came with great efforts; yet by slamming parts, or breaking Mattie's personal things to get a reaction from her was just ridiculous. The lengths Karen went through to make her angry was never ending. Belittling what Madison had accomplished made her feel quite relevant to some degree; she had Mattie watching her back. Nevertheless, Mattie kept quiet, but what happened next was unexpected as she slowly began spiraling in and out of focus in the heat of an argument, that leads to her breakdown.

It happened mid-morning sometime in late August 2003; it was close to school starting. The employee' s were waiting on their check's it was payday they all were talking about shopping for their kid's that morning, and how expensive clothing had gotten, it had to be around 9:15 or 10 A.M. when Madison received a call from the office inquiring Karen's whereabouts. Madison hadn't seen Karen all morning, because she had been moved to a new workstation temporarily. Madison told the secretary she had not seen the woman all day. This information got back to Karen causing rupture to her day. Right before lunch Mattie could hear Karen screaming at the top of her lungs as she sped closer to the area…("You are such a liar. You told my mother I wasn't working!) Mattie turned saying that is not what I said. I said …, I had not seen your stupid ass all day. Karen wanted to argue, call Madison names for the sake of a phone call. Madison tried to play past her antagonizing behavior, but couldn't. She put the paper work down to respond to the accusations, when she became lightheaded drifting in thought. Nothing was clear except wanting to grab her by the throat! Karen backed up, as Mattie got closer in what seemed to be a calm voice you need to get some help… something is wrong with you. Karen, continued shouting about her phone call keeping a distance between herself and Madison. Madison's thoughts blurred unable to respond right away, to what just occurred. A few seconds later, she felt this cool sensation drain from within dissipating from around her heart. It was silent as she turned away for a minute; …do something she thought. However, all she could do is walk to the women's restroom squirming to hold on to what little pride she had left to hold on to. It was too late she could not control her emotions from the stress of dealing with Karen. It had broken her mentally. Madison cried, and cried; because she let her spirit be broken" there was nothing left to fight with, only pain. A cold hollow feeling of powerlessness had come over her broken heart. Management was to blame for this disaster. Madison had written letter's accounting to Karen's behavior letting management know it had become a very unstable environment. Karen was so out of control that Mattie would not be responsible for her actions towards that woman. Management ignored the situation they reacted as if she was blowing the circumstances out of proportion by joking about Karen's antics with Madison' calling it a catfight" making light of her complaints. After that incident Madison became withdrawn in a since that all were invisible to her unless she had to acknowledge them. The work environment itself had major affects on Mattie's ability to function normally, or even focus for that matter. However, that lack of support for Mattie gave Karen the push needed to further her theatrics. This condoned behavior empowered Karen to abuse others, because there was no repercussion severe enough to deter her from acting hostile towards employees. Attacking others on the job was a way to get attention from management. This speaks to Mattie's point of her need to have recognition. Whenever, Karen acted out, all eyes were on her" swearing fiercely at whom ever made her feel inadequate' which was self-esteem issues really. Mattie went to work every day or as much as she could forcing down the fear of having to defend herself all the while continuing to question her own thoughts of rational. At the end of the day she was yelling at her own kids for stupid reasons such as leaving a glass on the coffee table, or a coat on the arm of a chair,.. later feeling awful about it. Madison soon recognized the anger inside stemmed from the work environment, and personal life not from her children. However, with that recognition of what she had been doing to her children the resentment towards everyone else got worse for taking the anger out on her children. Mattie became very belligerent at home mostly with her boyfriend for various reasons she lashed out eventually driving him away. His abandoning her said he really did't give a damn' about what she was going through, because he wasn't getting anything out of it. In the meantime while Madison was, falling apart 'work continued moving forward as if nothing were going on. It was killing her inside holding in all that hurt constantly apologizing for her actions at home, and at work. Yet Madison felt it necessary to hide the truth about feeling threatened all the time by Karen's mood swings. That fear of feeling trapped forced Madison to act irrationally lashing out at the questions of why the decision to keep quiet. Why"..You know damn well why. However, you go ahead keep your heads in the sand if it makes you feel better about what you're doing. Mattie seemed to be the only one having difficulties maybe even over imagining the incidents she's had with Karen. It was so bad; Madison nerves were shot further making her defensive of other co-workers motives for inquiring what her thoughts and feelings were regarding Karen. It was quite stressful on the job most days the fear in her head of co-workers plotting against her was causing her to switch into overdrive with the way management let that woman just run amuck 'getting away with harassing people for no reason other than she was miserable, which was despicable. Mattie resented having to look at Karen's face day in, and out with that intense feeling of expectation that seemed to gravitate from her sick mind. Karen just aggravated Mattie consuming her very soul unleashing a rage inside so unbearable it hurt. The idea of feeling forced to work with a mentally unstable person brought tears most days, but she just sucked it up and did what she had to do ... after all she had a family to support because she sure wasn't getting it from Jesse, he was too busy chasing after anyone that would give him what he wanted. Mattie put on a good face for all to see, but underneath was shattered glass held together by a thin skin. That following week accusations came out about, the way Mattie had treated Karen that brought about several meetings and one on ones to discuss work ethics on the job. Paul commenced to speak about company policy regarding the behavior on the job, and personal attacks there had been many involving that woman and because it was getting out of hand they decided to bring ethics into it stating , harassment would not be condoned. As employees, you did not have to like each other to get the work done. After hearing, his take on the situation Mattie felt it was necessary to deal with Karen more aggressively, because yet" ... again, nothing was done. It never was. Well there was that one time she went to counseling for drinking. That was just to cover her ass and to shut everyone up about the subject of her behavior. Why was she being so protected was beyond imagination. Karen's circumstances were more complicated than just being hostile as she confided in Madison and to others in one of her manipulative moments; that she was molested which forced her into a life of crime and a path of bad relationships. However, knowing about her past made confronting her even harder. Mattie's sympathy for Karen's trauma was forcing her to deal with the situation she was in delicately due to her state of mine. For Madison, this meant adorning a thick skin and getting as ugly, and combatant as possible to take the brunt of her attacks. Karen was known for nasty jokes or having someone else play cruel pranks on Mattie using any means spiders, dead rats, fake rats whatever would get a rise of Mattie. Karen's personality was so disturbing it was like viewing more than one person in a single moment. The woman had no morale ethics whatsoever it seemed, and she had no shiten-ass clue as to what that was. Karen was quite aggressive, and vindictive bent on revenge for her pain unknowingly unveiling herself to Madison for some odd reason. Yet, unknown and unsolicited Madison found herself the chosen one.

"Trapped in hell"

Madison found that she was slowly starting to run out of patients with Karen. The more stressed she became the more she spoke up facing Karen's crazy-ass' telling her she would not be controlling anyone in her area "not as long as she was in charge. Mattie thought about why she was taking on that responsibility, and if it were the right thing to do. Why was it her job? All she knew is someone had to block those attacks by Karen. No one deserved to go through what Karen was capable of dishing out. Madison had no other choice, but to become the wall to deal with Karen's strong personality she knew what the woman was like and had become familiar with some of her triggers. Karen was physical at times with other workers pushing them around to get what she wanted. It was uncalled for, and had happened more than once prior to the first attack. Stepping in at times was pressure on Madison to stay calm in her approach to the situation. This was not always easy to do. Approached by Vern, he expressed to Mattie that she needed to take a more aggressive approach in getting production completed, meaning she had to be forceful in her position as lead' thinking, for some reason they were getting comfortable with that hostile atmosphere created by her co-worker, who was quite sexually exploitive with her foolish performances, "yet mean spirited. Paul and Vernon seemed to be entertained at the approach. That would be understandable if it meant stepping it up in quantity, that is not what he wanted from Madison. He wanted a rougher more hardnosed approach. Madison refused to be rude or instill fear so those working would cower for their jobs. Refusing to follow their instructions garnered a standoff approach to her complaints regarding Karen. Of course, no one will admit to this, it is and has happened. The complaints were viewed as catfights, and disagreements as Paul, put it. Karen turned Madison's life upside down while reaping the satisfaction of gaining the upper hand. The disappointment Madison felt at the realization of being on her own told her all she needed to know. That the authority figure she had known no longer existed lost in a cloud of Kerens feel sorry for me manipulation cries. Management didn't give a damned about any personal problems she encountered with Karen, it was personal. Vern was responsible for insuring the safety of its employees and failed respectfully in doing so. As the supervisor, he should have written her up and given her a week's suspension or even fired the woman. However, with all the problems she complained about Management replaced Mattie, with another co-worker due to her ongoing lack of attendance, and failure to follow the procedures put forth, ultimately telling her in a subtle way that she could be replaced anytime. Unfortunately' Madison played right into Karen's desperate hands giving her the only possible advantage she could use to manipulate management in her favor "which was her attendance. That alone had become enough to give Vernon, and Paul something to use against Mattie. Fully aware of her attendance slipping had no bearing on what was actually happening to her mentally. Shit her attendance had slipped to an all time low something already known. Mattie' stayed home for any reason she could think of to avoid being in the presence of that woman; she has brought nothing, but hell and unnecessary problems to the job. She very much resented being used all those years as some type of buffer to allow those of you to slough off your responsibility for sake of entertainment. During those entanglements, Madison often thought she had a physical attraction to her what else could it have been to make her so combative. Mattie didn't know what to think or do? Her rude remarks to Madison's friends as they spoke with her were amusing at times, but what drove Madison crazy was her character changes between the episodes. Karen cursed Mattie for being silent around her stating ignoring her wasn't going to hurt her, but it did. Not even five-minutes later at the most she would be apologetic or even acting as if she never said a mean word to Madison. Madison could not figure her out to save her life. This woman had many sides to her twisted humor. Her pretense of not knowing what she had been doing to people sickened Madison to the point of slapping the shit out of her for playing silly ass games as a victim of abuse. The woman purposely manipulated people into giving her attention with her misfortune ultimately, allowing her to continue the spectacle she made of herself. Honestly, that pissed Mattie off! She was so blatant about her shit! She had aknack of playing the end against the middle. Madison could see what management failed to acknowledge, Karen knew this. A contagious illness we sometimes refer to as abuse by manipulation.,. Madison thought no other had ever witnessed the pain Karen was carrying around but there was another individual who had face-to-face encounters with her, and is the reason Mattie is dealing with her now. Finally, it didn't seem odd anymore that Karen would manage to turn her lack of attention into a work related issue when it was convenient. The scenario was easy create, …Madison wasn't helping her, she was supposedly hiding the work petty lies she made up when she was observed slacking on the job like she did all the time. Nevertheless, people were paying attention to her performance the girl had quite a talent for acting"... Madison often wondered what that was like for her.

This behavior forced Madison into acknowledging her presence whether she wanted to or not. It was more of a gesture on her part, and a necessity to protect others. Karen's moods were so up and down it was hard to approach the woman. She came at Mattie ready to complain and whine about the many difficulties she having to deal with. Management on the other hand, finally decided to do something about it; only after receiving complaints from other employees did they decided to send Madison to a seminar for managers. The seminar was about working with difficult and problematic employees along with her boss. What nerve; it wasn't her job to deal with that responsibility. However, she agreed. Madison made an effort to recognize others difficulties in getting along with those who are different. While it was quite heartening to be sympathetic after the mean things she had done over the years. Mattie always tried to turn the cheek, but when this tactic failed ignoring her was the best she could do without kicking that ass of hers. Taking responsibility for others, well being came natural; it was the right thing to do. Karen on the other hand has proven to be in need of medical help, and I am not a psychiatrist she felt responsible for the trouble Karen was causing for others who had to work with her. Understandably' she recognizes the anger and for this reason, Mattie had resentment issues for feelingforced to deal with such a burden; along with the lack of support needed to handle the situation. Yet, with Karen's volatile personality came hatred and disappointment for failing to maintain her part in that mess she erroneously participated in. Madison absorbed by the chaotic emotions in her heart to keep from feeling overwhelmed at seeing and hearing the pain of another which left her feeling there was no way out. Having no place to hide to release the weight was like drowning in tears of sorrow everyday for failing to live up to the persona she had come to know as her identity. Madison wasn't crazy' she knew exactly what was going on with her life she felt somehow that she was being forced to see the truth about self and life as it is. (Hell, helping this woman was not the problem. The problem was she did not choose this particular challenge" it fell into her lap. Maybe she was chosen," chosen to experience real suffering through the eyes of another… "to wake up and deal with her own personal denials about her family. Madison, laughed about it at times, because the efforts Karen made to get their attention was unbelievably misguided. Sex was always the weapon of choice for informing her co-workers of her personal encounters as to making them feel inadequate or less appealing to men than she were. The bosses praised her work; often giving her a false since of security in that she was very important to them, she even went as far as saying they were father figures to her in some respect. The point is she felt needed or valued. When Paul or Vernon turned her away she took, it personal for reasons unknown. However, the confidence management placed in Madison was fueling the tension between the two women. This angered Karen; that a boring woman who never spoke up about anything other than her children was blocking the opportunity for her to shine. Madison fed-up with Karen; went on a mission to save those in office from a walking disaster. These people were upper management; they had been hearing about the woman for years and a few had actually encountered some of her attitude having one man terminated over using abusive words towards her the same reason she should be fired. It forced Madison to go after her to get even by volunteering information regarding her behavior, and attitude on the job to a few of the supervisors in the sales department advising them to take a whiff of that breath of hers; that they needed no other evidence of her character besides the fact that she doesn't take criticism well. Simply stating she wasn't right for the job and her actions would speak for itself. This tactic was beneath Mattie; but all so necessary. Karen applied for a position within the company in the administration field passing some of the tests needed to qualify for the position, but another applicant had more experience than she acquiring the job. Karen Failed at being promoted, but wanted to know why. She started questioning others about her qualifications for the office position. No one said anything about what was mentioned only telling her to try for another when it opens again. Personnel' felt the other candidate was more qualified and more fitting for the position. Karen never stopped once to realize that people talk, that they might have heard about her actions and outlandish behavior on the job; it really stood out' the drinking, and bad attitude. This was just enough to do damage. Mattie was protecting them from her hidden talent to abuse, and attack for her own gratification. Simply pointing out how some folks can run their mouths just a little too damn much, failing to see the repercussions of their actions. Vernon was walking up to see Karen, after finding out she didn't get the job. Karen was expressing her disapproval of Madison socializing with the help to Paul, further stating her children were disrupting her workflow by calling every morning. Mattie turned away from what she had been doing, and proceeded to walk towards them to refute her claims warning Karen to back off. Karen had no idea of the work Madison had to do in the run of a day. Moreover, yes we all chatted from time-to-time with other workers as she had also unaware that Madison had arrangements to receive that 8 a.m. phone call from her child. The desperation for acceptance was forcing Karen to take whatever measure of action she could to get what she wanted "including aggressive behavior. As Vern interrupted Karen in the middle of her complaint, he proceeds to inform her of the news of not getting the job she applied for. Madison over heard, and had this smirk grin on her face snickering about what she had done. It was definitely the best news since deciding to quit. Madison hated whom she had become; observing the result of her actions after learning the position went to another. Karen went on a rampage shouting everybody hates her yelling, and snapping at all around her. Paul and Vern purposely avoided contact with her as much as possible. That anger Karen displayed made you want to run for cover. With the emotional baggage she came at you with you would think' she would get help. She thrived on tension; her sickness drove her to cause problems out of frustration. Karen made her personal problems so obvious that no one really wanted to get close enough to begin a friendship with her. The sense of jealousy truly comes to mind as she continued to demean Madison's character to get her to leave the job. Karen wanted to be the boss, to get it she needed to change a great deal about her character to appease management proving Mattie was to soft spoken, stuck-up, and stupid for refusing to follow the orders requested of her to be a successful in her approach as lead. Mattie didn't worry about what she said, because she didn't feel threatened by Ms. Filcher. Trusting in her own abilities as she have for the past six years of working there they knew what kind of person they had working for them. Mattie did not feel the need to be validated by anyone and wasn't afraid of any competition, especially from Karen. In fact' she was happy Karen had made every effort to compete for more responsibility on the job. It gave her something to focus on besides trouble. Madison was elated to see how much time she spent with Paul and Vernon" knowing she was up to no-good; it was fine as long as she stayed away from her. Although in the mornings she would notice them trying to escape her emotional outpours she greeted them with every morning' that woman could drive you crazy with all the shit she came to work with. At least they had somewhere to run. Nevertheless, for Madison it remained deep in her thoughts the questions of why Karen needed to be the center of attention all the time. Mattie summed it up as never having a stable relationship of any kind made her act out to get the attention she craved. The expectation of it frustrated Madison the most for tolerating a woman who has been misused, and abused to turn and disrespect women the way she does, and then react defensively to the criticisms of her actions. Was she that oblivious to her condescending behavior not to know what she was doing? Madison tried to help her sort through some of the reasons why she degrades herself the way she does having no shame about it. She looked so desperate at times when she spoke of her situation with men, Mattie iterated by telling her she didn't have to throw herself at a man to be appreciated. It was like saying don't drink water or something. In the mean time Madison never noticed how socially dysfunctional she had become. The challenges of taking on the responsibility of someone so ill willed affect how she reacted to all the difficulties in her life. Madison had been told several times by Louise, that she noticed the attitude change' she kept saying to her (girl you have to watch the way you talk to people). The tone you are using is too harsh). Madison didn't notice anything; this behavior had become the way of blocking out the hostility. (Really…, I sound mean.) Yes Mattie. Louise was right, I was rude and harsh, but for good reason and they will have to get over it. Mattie's emotions were all over the place working with that woman she is killing my nerves, and I'm jumpy always looking around to see if she is behind me,… now what kind of working environment is that. (Louise' the child is just not right") sometimes Karen stands five feet behind me staring not saying a word. That don't seem crazy to you. Look… Mattie you just gone have to ignore her the best way you can. Louise…" It's impossible. She is right there waiting all the time. It is unnerving to work with a person like that. You would be angry too… if you had to put up with her. As time passed Madison was fully engrossed in a mind battle of what her responsibilities were going to be. Her demeanor was constantly in play to accommodate the personality of a much rougher exterior I had taken on. It was, as if my body was aware of the negativity-taking place in my mind and my exterior was retrofitting the character personality of all the panic attacks, and defensive modes I adorned to meet the challenges faced. There were so many struggles being strong that I decided to confess what I had done. Although, I didn't want to, I had to clear my conscience it was the right thing to do. Madison walked over to Karen saying she had something to tell her, and it is going to make her angry, but she need to know, because she was tired of her constant badgering all the time. The reason you didn't get the job is, because I told those in office that it would be a mistake to hire you Karen, you are mean spirited, deceitful, and physically abusive to Lois and me for no other reason than jealousy. Karen, you said that about me. Of course I did. You do not deserve that position. Madison made it her business to stop it from happening. Mattie, told Karen she interfered for no other reason than to teach her a lesson in repercussions when you intentionally harass co-workers, spread rumors, and hit people to control them and that her behavior was intolerable to say the lease. Millicent, wanted her to know how angry she was about having to babysit a person with uncontrollable mood swings and changing personality. Karen was very upset by Madison's actions as she pondered what was said to her only to walk away mad. A few day's went by Karen wasn't talking. It was heaven for Madison. Karen was silent now that she knows everyone is aware of her behavior on the job. The drug and alcohol use went to another level, and her tantrums were more volatile. It became hard for Mattie to handle all her shit! The whole scene had Mattie on guard for her safety. She felt like the whole company was in on the sick joke Karen played. She had even gone as far as to spread a rumor about Madison and a co-worker. The rumor was that they were sleeping around Robert, heard it being discussed amongst the guy's, he alerted Mattie to this information and she lost her temper with the worker spreading this lie about her. Mattie, put down that tool walked down on the floor confronting Jeff to his face angry at what he was doing. You don't know what you're talking about spreading those damn lies. Mattie was shouting loud enough for everyone in the area to here she was so angry, That broad don't know shit about me as she fought back tears. Vern, walked up behind Madison as she got in Jeff's face, which was unlike her. Jeff was trying to tell Madison how Karen, had been telling them she'd been sleeping with her co-worker Robert a guy she worked with quite often everyone knew this Yet; he was only repeating what Karen had been saying about her. Mattie, thought for a man who thinks he is so talented in everything 'motherfucker, you sure were cheated in the intelligence department! The boss stopped the confrontation threatening to write her up forcing Madison to drop it as she stormed back up to her workstation still cursing mad. Nevertheless, the woman was mad about the rumor. She confronted Karen asking her did she say it, and she admitted to saying it with the biggest smirk on her face; as if it was her moral duty, wow Mattie, you can't even take a joke. Madison wanted to punch her in the face! However, she held back realizing this is what she wanted. Karen was on a mission to make Madison regret getting in the way of her possible promotion and refusing to associate with her. Madison replied (this isn't the way to gain friends girl. Her pride got in the way messing everything up. Karen's quite selfish and vein' she used her sex appeal to getting what she wanted manipulating people. Mattie thought this girl is just wild; don't you have any respect at all for yourself Karen? Karen would flirt, and act so sluttish with the guy's it was embarrassing. However, I do have to say; Madison envied her ability to just do what came to natural. For Karen the attention was far more important than the ideas of Madison's goody-two-shoe analyses. So Mattie' politely mentioned to management that she was finished. The reaction shown to her announcing she was leaving threw her off. It seemed as though they were expecting her to continue accepting the abuse, something they were willing to tolerate for the sake of production. That really didn't help Madison's state of mind' it rather made it worse. In that, her safety didn't concern them enough to look into her complaints more seriously. Madison felt she had been thrown to the wolves. Looking back, she realizes they did not intend to solve the problem, quitting resolved it. She just never realized how blind she was to what was going on. They weren't missing the point! In Madison's eyes it was the point, the catfight" it was what they had come to enjoy about the two of them, the fighting why else would a company allow such behavior. For her it went deeper than that. It was a question of stability, morals and your right to work in a safe environment. Madison's whole complaint was about safety. Management did not see to the work environment being healthy for everyone concerned. Madison didn't know where to go to explain the turmoil in this non-existent working relationship they thought was fine. Karen portrayed herself to be fine with all the hostility flowing from within. As Madison continued to pretend, she could handle it. It was pure negligence on their part to mishandle work place harassment, excusing it as just a misunderstanding. Karen wasn't happy; you could see this. It was as if she didn't want anyone else to be either. Madison slowly destroyed what was going to be her life. The sheer determination of manipulating others to hurt Madison was extraordinary to say the least. Madison sits at her desk thinking why this woman talks about her like a dog but wants to be in her face at all times wanting to talk about her miserable life trying to extract sympathy. "Who does this shit? It's something you'd normally see in a Lifetime TV episode") how aggressive is she going to get? Mattie's emotions were so out of control at times she would cry at the recognition of failure; a failure of realizing she had lost the battle and that her time was up. Focus girl! "Get your head straight. Here comes Vernon trying to making his presence known he is such a jackass the way he patronizes his employees. Hey Mattie, there is a meeting in the lunchroom now. Vern's arrogance was disgusting, but; she was going to attend that meeting. Madison has certainly had enough of the bull" this meeting was in regards to the havoc up in the work area which was "years to late if you asked Madison. Thinking finally" is the truth going to come out. Will she even tell the truth about her circumstances, and get some professional help or will she white wash it with more feel sorry for me stories. Paul interrupts' Karen as she voices her dissatisfaction of the work Madison does, I have no time for this you need to get along. (Karen mumbles under her breath), as Madison looks on staring at her pale skin and those bags under her eyes as if she hadn't slept in days; you know Karen it's not my job to hold your hand. Remember you're the super chick' it is what you want everyone to think, right. Always bragging about how much work you do! So do it. (Shut-up Mattie; "why should she, you don't want everyone to hear about your dirt. You know Vern Karen's attitude is just outrageous, she is pushy, insulting, and honestly, Mattie cannot tolerate the way she behaves. We are constantly accused of hogging up the work If Lois or she completes the work, if it takes longer, we are called names. Now who's crazy? Karen should be fired for attacking me, and everyone who tried to help her silly behind. The woman needs help! Mattie could feel this pull coming from Karen, a nagging feeling. To ignore her cries for help hurt Madison mentally, because the woman was suffering. Watching Karen, you could tell she had been through trauma. This cry for help was more than any one person could deal with. This is what slowly killed the spirit in Madison. That she could feel her pain. However, that hate was also taking over her judgment. She had come to realize that good faith speeches weren't the answer to the difficulties she was experiencing. A professional or therapist was needed the way she concentrated her rages on me. There was no way Madison could focus on the job all she heard was the sound of her mother's voice vibrating through her ears associating her voice with Karen's, which was intimidating enough by itself without the cord. Madison, forced to function as two personalities, one of a scared little girl who is afraid to say she is being hurt by someone else's inability to see they have a problem. The other is a wall of hatred and anger another voice inside her soul trying to escape from within to fight a real presence "one who is determined to bring her down. Madison, who lives in a made up world of everything is fine' is blocking this ability ignoring her personal problems as though nothing is wrong in her life, while all the baggage around her is slowly tearing down the walls around her. Living a non-existent life is what she knows. Learning to function as if the problems didn't exist was the way to survive the everyone's garbage. Her denial only helped to contribute to the damage she inflicted upon herself. By denying and forcing all the reality out of her head as she did as a child. Forced to be an adult at a young age you tend to forget you also exist when worrying about others. Madison never thought of her own needs before thinking of others there was no time for that. Madison is tired, tired of looking out for others especially those of you who never show appreciation. First, it was her siblings, that she didn't mind most days, then Jesse he doesn't get it, and now Karen who feels Madison beholden to her. What a fool she was, going through the motions of pretense has worn me down. There is nothing left to give. The pretense of having a happy home life has been hard on Madison and the kids; she is always upset at why Jesse refuses to help her with the kid's. Karen on the other hand nagged her for that same attention Jesse was running from. Madison wants to move on, but she will not get off her ass, and do it. What non-sense. Not recognizing he has worn her down to the bone dealing with his going to prison, and doing drugs most of their relationship. Only recently has she begun to really see Jesse for the person he has become, a self-serving cheating, and lying fossil of a man. Someone she allowed to keep her in constant defense mode to do battle. These thoughtless ungrateful beings reduced Madison to a shell of what she used to be. "I am not your mother" The pressure to be the leader came at an expense I was not prepared to pay. Expecting Madison to hold your hand, to solve the problems for others was more than she could ever expect to resolve on her own. Nevertheless, you kept taking and taking, advice, support even money she just did it thinking it would get better. It never did. Madison worked hard keeping that fear locked down, but unsuccessfully. Madison chose to play in a hostile environment causing me to become very abusive to the ones she love most. Madison had' had enough of the drama. What a fool she was to think that she could handle this mess. It had taken a toll on her spirit. Putting up a barrier to block the stress of others problems was how she chose to handle it. The innocent unaware of the devastation seem to suffer the consequences. For the first time Madison didn't have the answer to solve her own troubled life. Stupid for putting up with the garbage she has dealt with for so many years turned her into the evil person she was fighting. Real life, has been hard to take, and very overwhelming to recognize the seriousness of the problem. The fact that Jesse denies having an addiction and that there has been many times where there were signs she failed to acknowledge. During that time, she had not a clue as to what her sister was talking about when it came to Jesse, because she really didn't want to know or hear the truth. All she did was work, and take care of those kid's. Mattie closed her eyes to the rest of her life. The intimate part of Madison's life was about sex and nothing else the conversation was always one-sided. If there was anything nice to say, he always ruined it asking for money. When she did have something to say he would tune her out as usual. For the most part she felt Jesse was someone who could and would make a good man for any woman if he ever decided to change his circumstances. However, all she can think about is getting as far away from him as she can with the hope of starting a new life. These days it's shameful to say it aloud that she failed at having that life once dreamed. Today she finds her need to be there for others a detriment to who she could have been. Hiding behind others pain was a way to survive in her world where there was no substance or physical abuse. Especially when she herself has no real sense of what it is she is supposed to be doing besides picking up the pieces for others. Madison was totally committed to running from her problems with Jesse, and Karen. A force trying to extract from her the one thing she is unable to give. That shattered heart it was barely holding together it was cold and closed to any one asking of her. Millicent manifested off the hate boiling inside Madison's soul for letting them take part of what used to be her happiness, getting even with those of you who constantly hurt her while you feeing off her strength. If you abuse someone, enough they will snap out of fear there is nowhere else to hide. She felt like a moving target with a sign on her back misuse me. Mattie has been transparent for years even as a child. You could see her weaknesses, how to push her button's. Madison never shared her fears with anyone regarding the past except to her mother only bits and pieces after having the breakdown. Mattie asked her mother if she spanked them out of anger, because she had to raise them alone. No, Madison you were spanked because you were bad. Mom the way you looked when you were striking us was of enjoyment or some sickening desire to hear us cry out for mercy or something. Because you really don't have any idea of the fear, and pain you've caused for me and my siblings it's more devastating than you will ever acknowledge. Mom you know what you have done to us 'granted you stayed there for us. In my view, you resented being stuck with five kids and didn't hesitate to show it. Now Mattie is just like you mom resentful, and angry. The way you chose to chastise us caused a fear in my heart that has never gone away. Madison told you one time before that she was afraid of you, and it just missed you because you never listened or responded to that statement. "Madison feared you. Because, of this fear she never, ever spoke up for herself. Moreover, the last six years of her life has been devastating, because of "what might happen". Mattie could not defend the attacks from this woman Karen. The entire trauma that comes from an abusive relationship no matter the type can make' or break a person. With that recognition, Madison finally decided to get out by lying. Suppressing all that anger and hate stored in her heart was having an effect on the way she should respond to people. This role Mattie' was sucked into playing" is what she meant by feeling trapped. Madison regrets letting Karen walk all over her that way. She thought she was helping someone, now realizing she compounded the problem with all the resistance finding she was stuck in a bad situation. Was Madison supposed to take this abuse in order to keep her job? Because, it seems strange that her willingness to go along allowed for her to have some privileges that were not usually allowed which was the ability to arrange her time for personal obligations without questions or being written up things of this nature. Nevertheless, trying to relate with Karen failed, because her whole agenda was to manipulate and control. Obliging Karen" was a big mistake! Once she had the attention, she wanted Mattie, to continue holding her hand. Karen", continued to drink, having the same old complaint, of gaining control of her child. Now, what could Madison say to that? Telling her" (you get what you pay for; they laughed at her and behind her back. You cannot force a person to accept you; you have to learn to be patient for things to work out if she wanted her family back. She kept drinking, and acting a fool. Seemingly, she enjoyed the negative attention she latched on to more so than getting her self-stable. She thought with this responsibility maybe recognition would come in the future that never occurred. Madison got tired of the whole episode. She complained once again about having trouble working with the woman. Vern we don't get along, she keeps causing trouble with Lois and myself the cause is our unwillingness to hear her whine about her man. I am not interested in personal issues with her man. Karen had problems way beyond Madison's ability to handle; besides I am not trying to be a so-called baby-sitter to Karen. She behaved as if I owed her something. Always bringing up my kids as if she resented the attention they received from me. Madison didn't mind at times, but she didn't want to talk about her family with Karen, her interests were insincere. Mattie was feeling pressured for her time" it was too over powering to the point' of a harassing type behavior. The family acceptance Karen was seeking is what drove her continued need to grab at others. Madison stayed angry with her because of the constant neediness' coming from her. She is attacking the wrong people for what is missing in her life. Madison opened her heart to a predator, and she cannot protect it any more. With three kids" the choices alone made her angry having to choose between a roof, and food" or sanity. Emotionally torn inside about not being strong enough to fight has made her very critical, and untrusting of anyone. They proved Madison right in her thoughts of them while being escorted from the building. The pain Madison holds is from abuse obviously. A face of make believe, and denial to what life is like. She resented all of you for destroying that place for her. No one has the right to cause another pain for his own gratification, or lack of. First, my confidence was gone. Madison wasn't sure about the suspicions she had about the supervisors if they were plotting against me, and if they let everything happen because they wanted me out. Madison's thought's were so out there it was hard for her to tell what was real and what wasn't "it's sad. Mattie lived in a dysfunctional state of mind, and created a life within a life. Madison couldn't even begin to tell you all the things that happened right in her face never once acknowledging it until the breakdown. Madison separated the two worlds that she lived in for over twenty years. She just wanted to be happy. It was just more lies she told herself to feel good inside. Foolish thinking, she must admit; however, inside that tough exterior Madison was honestly dying inside. It couldn't get any worse for her. Some days all she did was cry at work even while typing the emotions were so powerful, because she felt trapped. Not one person could see the hurt in her heart having been this strong entity for so long. It felt like she had taken on the worst challenges any one person could handle. Madison ultimately had become a different person than who she was inside. Having splinted into different personalities to function, speaks to how bad the stress was for her. She seemed to be shutting down, while the inner personality was taking over. The ability to reason was more of a vengeful personality in essence. Keeping her under control wasn't easy. It took everything' I had inside from falling apart in front of everyone. Holding back the emotions and tears slowly broken her down, because of all the pain suffered. Madison was clueless as to what to do; she could trust no one to help her. All I ever heard was, we all have problems girl 'just deal with it. Madison tried to deal with the problems for a long time, but how do you handle problems that are not yours, but somehow have become yours. Mattie put herself out there for others and now Mattie carry a rage so deep it has become what I am today. Was the hostility really happening as she thought it was, or was she losing her mind. Can it be that she is the only one to see what's going on with Karen? How can this be Mr. Jenson? Thomas Jenson normally would have been working on rigs a mechanic for twenty-five years was helping catch up with the load that day because, work was slow for him that week. While working on paper work we heard a commotion around the corner Karen shoved Lois into some freight for not working fast enough for her and Lois shoved back! (Jenson, said look at her laughing" how do you put up with it? Madison said yeah! She knows. Mattie just reported her, and he laughed thinking it was Lois, who told on her, because it was Lois originally attacked by Karen, not Mattie. Madison was sick of it (Vernon he wasn't doing anything about our situation it was like' who cares. So Madison went over his head' something they don't like you to do. There were no other choices. (Mattie was still grinning from turning Karen, in to personnel and a long waited decision to quit gave a since of relief even if it was temporary. The headache of trying to refrain from beating her down was just about all she was able to do to keep from putting her hands on the woman. Mentioning this to Vernon was like talking to a wall. She got nowhere. "It was one of many episodes' just like this one, but this time she was ready to walk out! The rage was so intense there was nothing stopping Madison from killing her. Just to see her hands on that girl's throat gave promise to a well-earned piece of mind only to give way to Madison's nagging pull not to touch her! (Grab that bitch Millicent! (Karen was pouring it on'

28

the disrespect, and loud accusations steadily trying to humiliate her pushing her to the limits for going to personnel to report what she had done to Lois and myself. Madison was the only one working up in the area, although frank was in the shipping office, Millicent' wasn't sure if he could here Karen shouting at her). Usually they would stand watching in amusement, not this time" it was just (Karen, and Millicent" face to face. Millicent was leaning over a cart' with a rage burning so deep, she was ready to bash her head in right then. The only thing separating us was plastic curtains. But as usual; Madison's conscious prevailed, or failed' depending on how you look at it, which is how she saw it' smiling, and gritting her teeth, thinking she can't continue doing this, it hurts so much. Madison lets the tears run in silence' as she continues working. How much longer will I have to endure this hateful ass woman?   Karen was moved from the area. The excuses for being there were ridiculous' saying it was for her phone call one of her many ways of being in Madison's face with her shenanigans. But on this particular day there was a calm feeling in the air to the point that Madison was feeling ok. The next day she was working fine' It was so pretty outside' a fresh baked smell was blowing through the bay doors from the bakery across the street and I was quite busy getting packages ready to ship the music played aloud it made the day go faster. Watching Ms. Karen, flashing to some of the more colorful character of people she has portrayed. (I, knew she was unaware of acting out at her inability to cope with her insufficiencies' by the words coming out of her mouth, and it probably would remain that way unless she sought help. Look we all have an associate, or two in our lives that we have to deal with just on principle, who aren't wrapped so tight, but we tend to be able to laugh at the "humor in it all, but in her case it was nothing to laugh at. Laughing" was another way for me to handle dealing with her. Sometimes you want to laugh while wringing her neck. At the same time I was falling apart trying to front I had it under control. but deep down within was a thin line between sanity and insanity' losing control of what used to be a soft spoken person that did not mind lending a shoulder to others now in a paused state of mind viewing her self-destruction. Something is very wrong with you! Seriously" Millicent appeared to Karen, if you don't step off, I will hurt you girl. The emotion flowing was raw, and unreal. The sensation was as if nothing else mattered in those few moments" all I saw, was "Millicent, picking up a part to crack her in the mouth. She wanted to shut her down to make her feel the loss of existence she had taken. Still the satisfaction of whooping her ass was much more tempting, and possible But it never happened' something else happened.

Chapter 2
Unstable Behaviors

"Stuck with the Demon from Hell"

Karen was observed on many occasions banging parts on tables and slamming tools to get attention, which wasn't an ideal job for Madison. The idea of having to massage Karen's emotional scars was ludicrous. All I wanted to do is choke the shit out of her, and take a cigarette break in celebration for silencing her crazy ass for a least a moment" and for the guts to stand-up to her unlike those who were in charge. Just a thought'... since choking the woman wasn't an option without going to jail. Madison continued working as if nothing bothered her by creating, some distance between herself and the plethora of unsettlement that always followed. I did what was necessary to make folks who were unaware of Karen's hidden talent to attack every opportunity to be prepared for their own safety. Mattie dealt with her for years obviously obliging her ridiculous need for attention so she knew what to expect from her "although she preferred she see a damned psychiatrist! Madison was tired of her. Nevertheless, the reality was... Madison accepted the behavior from Karen for years feeling an obligation for volunteering to work with her. This was not my job; I had problems of my own at home with my children's father who also had serious problems. He had the opposite effect on her at home. Madison had become the aggressor in a fight that felt like there was no end in ight. I wanted to quit my job several times, but the idea of quitting made her feel like she was running out on her responsibility. Moreover, Madison would be giving up all the time she put into making that position her own. Knowing she had used all her sick leave and vacation time pretty much left no options, but to quit. Reluctantly Madison lied about the reasons fearing that telling the truth about her situation would make them think less of her. She did not reveal the source of her true pain of feeling responsible for two adults who were addicted to drugs and alcohol, and apparent mental problems. They had no idea of the destruction they were committing' Karen's tirades of anger perceived by most in the shop were hilarious and crazy acting, but not one person working there wanted to trade places with me. The last employee she worked with had Karen removed from his station. He had experienced some serious difficulties in communication with her. Karen had a trash mouth that wold give the hardest hardcore trucker a run for his money" she was just nasty. Nobody ever mentioned why she was moved to production until several months later. By then it was too… late. Mattie had absorbed her emotional baggage stuck working with her for weeks on end subjected to the daily ritual of having to endure the un-pleasantries of being in her company.

"Looking for acceptance in the wrong places"

Karen was in need of serious medical attention, as she continued functioning inebriated on a fulltime basis to dull the connection of anger to the truth of her destruction. This woman had deep scars and unhealed wounds that told many stories by her actions that were killing her inside. Oblivious" to what she was doing to others. Karen was looking for that forgiveness or acceptance from the innocent souls and fools unaware of her true face except for Madison who saw right through all the hostility. Madison sometimes noticed her sitting at her worktable staring steadily with those angry eyes; it was as if she was trying to make Mattie disappear or something. Acknowledging her antics, Madison felt she could manipulate the situation to a better atmosphere for both of them by taking an interest in some of her concerns about the relationship and abuse, and abandonment from family to ease the tension. Reluctantly Mattie, allowed Karen to be a part of the planning and decision-making to keep her from talking about the personal part of her life, which seemed to bring out the worst in her. None of that worked, because as soon as she agreed to listen to Karen they never got anything done. All she ever did was whine about her boyfriend, or her mother and what they had done to her. Please, I can't hold your hand. Madison found it quite hard to keep up the charade of strength, for which had devoured into hopelessness in her heart while struggling to keep her own family together. How could this happen allowing herself to be sucked in between two lives that were broken by circumstances she had no control over Karen, who was desperately seeking help, and Jesse who was trying his best to hide. Jesse was her man for better or worse they met through an acquaintance at his apartment in October 1984, a young man who came across as a kindhearted soul, who made her laugh, but always on the go. Jesse was never a man of expression he mostly just did what he had to do to survive. He didn't have much of an education dropping out of school his junior year, but his Mechanical ability could have given him a great career in the blue-collar industry. I told him this all the time not sure, if he listened. The man could fix just about anything on a vehicle. When he worked, he appeared confident in himself during those times. It is when he is not occupied in complex work that he'd drift away from his family. Jesse is a fine man, and over time, she convinced herself he could do anything. Through the years, she allowed the attention she got from him to dilute what was in her face all the time... the addiction. He appeared to come from hard times as she had. Madison thought they had a chance to overcome any obstacle yet' there was this constant need to be in the streets. Madison never questioned where the money came from because she worked and did not depend on him for sole support at least financially. It wasn't until much, much later when she finally realized he had the addiction, by then it was way too late. This information only made it harder for Mattie to force him out because I knew there was more to the story than what was being shown. Madison's relationship was so one-sided it was bound to crash with all the burdens falling in her lap. Things were rough at home, as she began to change in character to address her anger at his inability to help out. She too…was damaged goods, but well painted and versed. How was she going to inspire another to seek help when she had her own nightmares, and skeletons? That fear of getting in trouble stayed on her mind when dealing with these two. Mattie worked alone with this woman forty hours a week for almost ten years in close quarters hearing the anger spilling from her mouth for six years and counting. That constant rage locked Madison down. Speaking up wasn't part of her character. That ability halted by all the beatings received as a child that previously shut her down as a child. The association between the two instances was more than enough to drive a person to close up, but she kept trying by confiding a little of her own personal background regarding family issues with drugs, and abuse thinking she would finally get it that Mattie was not the enemy. Nevertheless, Mattie sits on the other side of this battle feeling trapped by the inability to speak her mind. That presence of anger filled the air "it felt as if she were at home again like a scared child waiting for a whooping for something she couldn't control. A familiar atmosphere she buried deep in the back of her closet. It was eerie at first to feel that same stillness that silence she felt as a child. I would get scared then mad about the fear coming back afraid to move at times afraid to speak up. (What a joke.) Mattie kept quiet about the pain and stress she held in for years due to the mental stress Karen caused making her a silent part of Mattie's job. Since know other seemed to care about the two women's dilemma Madison played the game best she could to survive the mess she slowly sunken into eventually pushing her to relive her own scary past as they inter-twined with each other. Madison decided to let her guard down for what was going to be her chance to show them she could be a positive team player, and role model yeah a role-model, please…, this chick needed help) a therapist she wasn't. Madison had always been sympathetic to others for as long as she could remember having been through some of the toughest situations a child could go through. (Yet' sometimes it felt as if she were reliving her childhood fears once again. The battles with Karen took her back to being berated by her mother. Instead of seeing Karen, it was her mother's image surfacing; this vision prevented Madison from acting out her urges to retaliate. Mattie couldn't risk anyone knowing about that fear. Determined not to let them see her shattered spirit walking in the shell of which she once was. I pretended to be focused on my work unable to decide who I should be or how to act. Her thoughts blurred constantly thinking about what to do about her troubles with Karen. In the midst of a crisis, Madison took many vacations and sick days off to get away from Karen unable to hide the pain only to lash out at her children. For Mattie to continue looking past all the insults, and attacks on her person was ridiculous. The lack of support shown in her situation made controlling the urges to be violent impossible. The possibility of doing harm to Karen in her state of mind was forcing Madison to fight her own rages of anger for the attacks all those years.

"Changing Faces"

They were too… stupid to see past their own noses the destruction-taking place in this woman's mind. A woman who needed them to recognize the signs lashing out, yelling all the time, the fact she only takes pride in her work when she is shown gratitude, but that was the exception. Karen was manipulating, conniving sneaky person that became quite combative to get her way. Unable to see there was a woman in need of serious help. Karen wasn't some devilish entity that just happened to come after Mattie, not at all. Karen was quite lost looking for something, or someone whatever it was Mattie felt like she was seeking it from her with all her outrageous commotion. To describe Karen, she was a nice looking woman with shoulder length dark wavy hair; skin pale looking, and her eyes stayed puffy probably from the alcohol or lack of sleep. Her eyes were light brown glaring with suspicion all the time. Karen was suspicious of the boss talking with Madison from time to time about the week's shipment, and expectations for the day, which was fine for the most part. What these observations of Karen showed me was to stay alert. Karen could be pleasant enough to be around if you danced around the personality changes, she adorned throughout the day. What made working with her so difficult was she thought; somehow, Madison was plotting against her with the bosses. This was not the case and from then on life on the job became hell for Mattie. One thing for sure there was no respect between the two entities. Karen pretended to be nice on the surface for those she hid her pain from, yet; always willing to reveal her true face when it suited her needs. What Madison felt was this deep pull coming from Karen as if; to will attention towards herself a need she constantly craved as though she could not function without it. However, Madison found that some of us tend to hide the sides of our selves we like to keep hidden from the world for reasons we care to forget "until that one single incident or moment in our lives forces it to reveal itself as I had come to do.

"Working With Sybil"

Thinking on it; Madison should have quit her job years ago, but it wasn't in the cards. Quitting her employment with other obligations weighing in on her decision was not a choice she could make at that time. This made her life very difficult keeping in mind she had children to take care of that needed a roof over their head, and food in their mouths. Madison always refused to let that Demon run her away, not to be the one to give up the fight for what was right. Observing her it looked as if; she was making an effort to control her anger. Now I knew better than that, Karen could play a part as good as some actresses I've seen as she made her rounds gossiping about me, and how lazy I happen to be with any who'd give an ear. The behaviorisms Karen displayed; it really had taken her back especially hearing her admit aloud that she told some of the men in the shop the reasons they were absent on the same day was, because they were lesbian lovers. They would laugh in curiosity as to why she behaved as if; she didn't recognize the seriousness of her actions. What's even more astonishing' was her facial expressions of being unaware of what she had been doing. The woman was just different as she glared at the bosses private parts snickering about the sizes of their manhood. Madison wondered where she had been working before coming to work for this company. There is no way a credible company would tolerate this behavior. Karen felt Madison walked around as if her shit doesn't stink, always looking down her nose. Karen couldn't stand her pretending to be above drama, and problems of everyday people. Bothered by her ability to leave personal life at home seemed to easily set her off yelling at other workers for doing a job she may had intended to do, or for saying hello" to a passerby. It rubbed her wrong no one comes to work without something to complain about. It was enough to make Karen kick rocks what a mess.

"Lashing out"

For the past two years, it has been nothing but mistakes looking back at all the signs that were left for me to see. Trying to appreciate all of the hardships gone thru, and those she has yet to go through brings tears to her eyes. Just looking back on all the episodes made her want to scream for putting herself through that hell. Today, name-calling is Madison's choice of abuse these days when it comes to expressing whatever is wrong with the child" especially if her point isn't taken seriously. For years she's sat in the shadow letting others use her as some type of squeegee. Well that time has come and gone, you can't shut her up! Everyone was to blame for her downfall. Jesse the reason for her failures had become the main target of her verbal abuse, how could he have cheated on her, and left her while she was at her worst. The only thing he cared about was what he could squeeze out of her. She gave that man the best of who she was as his woman and threw it in her face, as if she didn't matter to his black ass anymore. With every thought of betrayal he committed against Mattie, she finally had the nerve to tell him exactly what she thought of him and his spineless ways, you ain't shit, and you will never amount to anything for what you have done. Madison changed morally in behavior the things she prided herself for caring about no longer mattered. The surroundings and situations played a major part in the separation of mind, and spirit. Waking up in rages, from the expectations of being harassed, made for a very sad and angry person.

Chapter 3
The Breakdown

"Where was the control?"

Understanding fully' why people use the term" (Madison was broken up by this overwhelming feeling of failure as she drove home in a frozen state of mind' what just happened? Why didn't I knock that woman on her ass? I wasn't afraid of her all it would have taken is just one blow, that's all. I still could not touch her. Mattie's head was spinning out of control feeling distraught by everything that had taken place that week. Her son had been in a car accident, he survived thank goodness, and she found her so-called man out with another woman. It couldn't get any worse than knowing I allowed it to happen. I made the decision to let him drive the car which was my fault. Then if that wasn't enough she found her man driving another woman around in his car. The woman was surprised and quite nervous grabbing her belongings as I leaned into the car grabbing the woman by the arm proceeding to pull the woman out of the car, when he comes running with his sorry ass" (Mattie! he says, what are you doing? As if, she was the one out of pocket or something. Who in the hell is this bitch, Jesse? All the Bastard could say was just go home Madison, (I'll be there. as he jumped in his car making that quick exit from embarrassment. Mattie felt foolish in her behavior it was so beneath her to act a fool in public or elsewhere for that matter. The first thing I noticed after the scene was a security camera, I was being recorded how stupid I must appear. Madison realizes it wasn't the woman she should've been trying to beat down 'it was Jesse's ass she should've gone after.

Maybe' it was her last ditch effort to stand-up to the wrong in her life. Madison felt betrayed by all in her life. It seemed as if every person there at the gas station had eyes on her. Madison would not have sunk that low as to confront him that way if she were in her right state of mind. Now if she isn't mistaken a few weeks prior to this incident she made him move out, because he was staying out all night, and trying to convince her he wasn't cheating. However, he's only been gone all of a couple of weeks, and already sleeping around or had been apparently. Mattie felt her accusations were true, although he denied it. This was a man she has been with for over nineteen years, a man she has gone through hell and high water with, and for what. Mattie stood by his broke ass during all his down time. Most would say her stupidity allowed him to do this, but for me being stupid has nothing to do with what he does in those streets. I refuse to be a babysitter to something I knew was mine. I know this man loves me no matter how ungrateful the son of bitch seems to be. I am a woman, not a girl so to run every time my man fuck's up, say's a whole lot about my ability. For one I don't have to join them to beat him at his own game I just had to figure out what to do. Jumping on the first man willing to do you the favor was not an option especially when I knew he loved me. Madison stood by her man in all instances, even when he was in trouble. Yes, I was angry, but I got over it, something we have to keep the family strong for all it was worth. For him it was retaliation for her past indiscretions') yet; no matter what he has faced and beyond, Mattie was his main supporter. The betrayal was just too much to absorb. After that incident, things just started falling apart. Mattie never realized that being morally responsible could be a reason to betray someone. While everyone else around her went on with their lives and having a good time. She was suffering emotionally she just was no match for the turmoil ruining her life. "Thinking, she was such a fool? After being so vigilant in standing her ground, she had actually lost the battle! How can this be? How could she be so giving and supportive to others in her world only for them to triumph over her? Was it possible for someone so angry and hateful to be able to triumph over another who was kind hearted and gentle in handling any situation to be misused and abused the way she had been. Well we now know the outcome, with all the misfortune and bad luck, Madison never dreamed she would be homeless and broken as she is today. The self-respect and dignity was gone. She totally became non-existent in an non-existent world. Afraid to move forward with her life, because she fears there is only hardship ahead. Afraid she will have to give something up of herself has begun hiding in fear of having to indulge in conversation. A fear had taken over her ability to socialize with strangers; hello for her meant having to respond in kindness something she could not do closing up like a coward out of fear for trying to do the right thing. The heartache of finding out the truth about her manifested reality brought an ugly side to the unknown person she had become. However, why was the pretense so harmful to others when doing the right thing was her only motive in life? Why Madison felt she would be viewed negatively in a society, because the way the world seems to be revolving "is that if you aren't about taking, then you are perceived as a loser, or stupid for not expecting something in return. Sometimes the return is not about what you have done, it's about the accomplishment of doing it. She believed in something taught to her as a child, destroyed by a few individuals in a matter of a few years. However, those of you who look at being a good person" as a sign of weakness and stupidity' are shall I say greatly disturbed, at best un-happy with self.

Madison's unwillingness to taking a more vigilant approach to the situations she was facing with Karen who did appear the more dominant of the two was in fact quite intimidating. Madison didn't want to take matters into her own hands, by physically hurting the woman like she wanted to; it wasn't going to solve their problems. Never the less Madison wanted her to suffer the way she was. The vengefulness" It wasn't who she was in her heart. The anger was totally an entity in Millicent's world, (Madison was and has always been calm and quiet, but as you can tell, she had changed. Feeling she is and has always been seen as a pushover in the eyes of those she trusted. Not making "Karen" regret what she had presumably caused Madison and her family to live with. Ultimately that is what she wanted' to see Mattie's pain making it possible to gain control. It wasn't the job driving her hatred of Madison. Karen was trying to get control of her own miserable life with selfish motives. This attempt became a problem for Madison Karen was trying to go through her to prove she was as much in control of her life, as Madison seemed to be. She made a point to assume hurtful things about her boyfriend Jesse, thing's she had no knowledge of being true or not! If Madison seemed too… confident in her relationship with her man it was, because she chose to live as if; it wasn't any ones damned business. Moreover, has been the case the last six years they've worked together up until the day of quitting. To recall a day when Madison had control of her outcome she would almost have to be in a psychosis state of mind. The depth of the situation had taken a toll on her, as she would become unable to control her personal feelings of betrayal, "stabbed in the back helping them out! Why should Mattie cry on the shoulders of the ones who created this disaster? The same people who encouraged Mattie to be more sympathetic to a woman who played a big part in her destruction. Karen was allowed to wreak havoc whenever she pleased forcing Madison to defend herself.

They could not see Karen's problems were deeper than what was visible on the surface. They barely sneezed at the commotions taken place up there in the warehouse. By making Madison aware that she was replaceable at anytime by putting Lois in her position to control her ability to dictate her authority. Taking her position away was a way to teach her a lesson, but allowing Karento get away with being high or even inebriated was tolerated even ignored. The supervisors never saw her drinking, or doing drugs, but they could smell her a mile away, "that is the same thing. They knew Madison was angry about having to work with Karen mentioning it in many ways. Neither Lois nor I wanted to work with Karen she was a tyrant. Some employers fail to realize tat its one thing to be a team player it's another to be an all out security guard for their employees. I felt exactly that way. When you are working and with the same folks everyday you tend to have a connection with them and for those I did know for a long time deserved to work in a safe environment. The tolerance of Karens' excessive abuse brought forth the worst anger Madison had ever felt causing her to have emotional outpourings, because she felt held back by her physical capacity to whoop her natural-ass. Sure Mattie could have just gotten physical with Karen, she has tried many times at pushing her to the point of violence" praying was all she could do keep from seriously blasting her in the mouth, but what good would that do? She would go to jail loing her job" then what? Karen could run rampant on any and all who comes her way. I wasn't having it! The little games people of power like to play to keep you in line can be exhausting to a do gooder like Madison , yet it seems to have no ending". Madison realized' she created some of the problems, but it was the only way for her to block all the drama going on at the time. Attendance was the last thing on her mind, her sanity was at stake, and only she could salvage it by being guarded. It also proved that she wasn't capable of handling someone with these severe emotional problems, which she stated repeatedly. How could it have turned out any other way than it did with management refusing to see the problems for what they were? Madison was an emotional wreck from fighting to keep her sanity. Every day she had to come up with a way to sustain the hysterics' she endured daily as they went about their business as usual. Wake up girl! This isn't pretend" your life is falling apart in front of your eyes. Madison was so emotionally drained by all she had taken on that running away from all her troubles was looking like her only escape. Contradicting her practice of resolve now, rather than later was looking more appealing as time passed living as if it didn't exist. Acknowledging that Karen's presence in her life had brought to life all the darkness she managed to bury years ago. A woman torn inside with agony and hate the opposite of what Madison was in spirit she whole heartedly hid none of her pain; it was there for all to see, "in fact forcing Mattie to deal with her own anguishes, and choices in life. Even as a kid' she was too afraid, fearing that no one would listen to her cries for love. The need to be heard or understood to this day remains as she continues to search as she struggles to reconcile with her downfall. Madison recalls one summer day long ago, as she sat with her oldest son's father talking about the baby she gave up, and why. Mattie never responded to his questions because it wasn't her choice to not have that child' that was decided by her mother, unwilling to speak her mind she ignored the questions instead. He Said to her quite angrily ("one day girl all the shit you keep bottled up inside is going to kill you. If you don't start talking about it, "it's going to eat you up inside"). At that time, I was only sixteen years old, and didn't give his comment a second thought' because I was more concerned at what he was trying to do by acting as if he cared that I hadn't had the child he was so busy screwing any who allowed him to it was a joke?   All she thought he wanted was to take something from her"… to know what her private thoughts were. Mattie had nothing to say that would be even remotely interesting to him, or anyone else to speak of that would interest them in getting to know her personally. There was no substance; no reality to speak of in a since, because she hadn't discovered who she was at that time, Besides no one ever listened to Madison "not really; especially those who could have guided her in a positive direction. Go play; is what she were told. That child couldn't have anything relevant to speak of is what they said. First of all Madison was to shy, and too quiet for most. Do you see why it was so easy to take advantage of a person like Madison, she was good at being seen and not heard. Mattie learned to deal with pain by keeping it inside. The wounds never healed from being denied her identity, and the cries were never heard; not even by her Mother which made speaking up pointless. The yearn for answers started a long time ago, with this deep seeded need to find her father a man who abandoned her long ago leaving her to fend for herself and her siblings. The man never appeared not even for his own daughters' funeral. This man allowed her to believe he hated her, and that the reasons for his abandoning her were true. It hurt us kids to know that we had a father who could just up, and walk away from five kids, and start a new life with another and raise her kids that were not his so easily. Madison never got over that rejection, and her family never made it easy to forget how her father didn't want her. What kind of family does that to kids?   Where was the example? I saw this bending over backwards from my mother and grandmother to please' how was I to know that it was ok to say no! To speak my mind "if I did not want to be used or taken for granted wasn't not tolerated. I never saw one of my elder women family members speak out against it. It was like a passing of the foolish torch being transparent to the world exposing her deepest fears, and weaknesses, but most of all the desire to be free from everyone, her brothers, and sisters is what kept her motivated to hold on.

Madison hated living in fear" it was and has always controlled how she made all her decisions, always thinking that if she did only what she wanted, she would be viewed as selfish, and thoughtless and more so disliked not by just family but mostly everyone that came into contact with her. Expression of self has been a problem for quite some time she must admit, and stepping up to the plate when push comes to shove was always scary. So many of her decisions were made out of fear it's a wonder she has made it this far. The fear of speaking up ruined the freedom she could've had in all that mattered to her. The choices in life' the man in her life, where she lives and the type of career paths taken lead her where she is today are some of the choices she regrets. There is so much more inside this chained up heart if she would only open the door just a little "who knows what the possibilities are and only she can expose the real woman inside?

Chapter 4
The Blame

"You failed to see it coming!"

Invisible 'that it was… for Madison not to see what was in front of her, but only that to which fitted her needs was an accomplishment. For it is the trap she set for herself repeatedly. Growing up the oldest kid it was only natural having to be a caregiver something she was not to be ashamed of. All families have siblings who take care or help with responsibilities with Madison though she had taken on another form of that responsibility. Her mother did it, and her grandmother cared for others. Yet' to embrace difficulties without discouragement or complaint displays a whole other side of our character being… for it is what makes her special. Madison has always known this to be her personal talent, but has never really taken the time to look at it objectively wondering why it was so easy for her to reach out to others in need before thinking of the consequences. The warnings were never clear to her, but most definitely left signs, or feelings of weakness and gullibility. Mattie read the world as a giving and kind atmosphere by seeing only what she chose to see in any scenario setting herself up for serious letdowns. How do you walk away from one in need of help? I never claim to be anything other than self, a friend, confidant, and supporter if it were asked of me I just gave. This woman confided to me some of her most painful experiences, because I made myself available to her. To be kind is not a crime, but taking ones kindness for granted should be. Treating one less than for refusing to conform to their selfish, mean spirited ways told me they had been mistreated at points in their lives. No wonder she had no clue as to her own identity... with arms open to all she was unable to think of self, because she had so many hands to hold. Madison had no life without the problems of others to keep her focused. Mattie never heard of self identity… 'which she now realizes was the ultimate reason for her demise as she continued setting herself up for emotional letdown. What was self-identificationwhat did it had to do with me. The time had come to accept life for what it is. A beautiful growing vessel of destinations and sprawling paths leading to, but not excluding heartache, misconceptions and desperate cries of exceptions where desperate people will stop at nothing to take what you have, sometimes at great costs. This hurt tremendously to think that all you are worth to others is what they can drain out of you. There was no appreciation for the time lost out of her life. Taking the blame for what was happening was enormous in itself, because to blame Karen who truly had no idea of what she had accomplished in her desperation for acknowledgement could hardly grasp Madison's destruction. Mentally she destroyed the spirit that made Mattie the kind person she once was "becoming yours and our worst nightmare. Now a replica of what she despises finds herself in a battle of wills with a side of herself she refuses to acknowledge in her search for compassion and the ability to forgive. Mattie didn't want to let go of the rage that kept her so depressed and miserable. Why would she do that! There was no satisfaction in letting go' I had to make them feel like I did …thrown away, how's that for stubbornness. The pure selfishness of those she has given her heart to seem to walk this earth as though their miraculous ability to thrive successfully came about all on its own. To acknowledge their true colors would be a difficult task as she tries to find a sense of balance in her life. Internally hating what has become her reality, __ a mirror of what has been the opposite of a woman that loved unconditionally without judgment.   Those of you who have taken pleasure in destroying that graciousness, in which she once possessed of course, will refuse to acknowledge the involvement in creating the hardened and pained person you see today. There is nothing, but anger and mounds of questions. Karen's lack of appreciation for Madison's participation in her new found ability to show she had the ability of forgiving within the deepest part of her damaged soul her pretense of a life we now see in her demeanor at times. Thus far brings to question some of the goodness happening to her was it Mattie's involvement that undoubtedly influenced some of (Karen's not so quite, obvious good behavior. Madison tends to believe this to be true. Yet; to this day only resentment has been able to survive in that heart of hers towards Karen and everyone who took part in the destruction of a kindhearted fool. Tired of feeling as if she was a rug to be stepped on Madison got angry taking matters into her own hands. By accepting responsibility for the destruction of her failed life as it was she decided to put her life together one day at a time? Quitting that job was the beginning of what was to be a hard fought and cried out recognition of self discovery. First working on the anger, she had to lose that hostility towards people. Mattie went on a feel sorry for herself trip by blaming lack of support for her plight on family, that ungrateful man of hers any and all she could to excuse her spiraling downfall into drug use' who cared… she thought. Why not do it everyone else did Madison didn't feel the need to be better than the rest in her eyes people loathed do-gooders such as herself. Now unemployed about to lose her apartment allowed another to give her crack" she hit an all time low. Pretending to be in control of her actions while getting high her man was all too willing to assist… he had found a way to get his high on through Mattie, when she was at her worst point in life. Madison needed him to support her at the lowest point in her life"… and he only took advantage of it. He manage to talk her into getting high by preying on my vulnerability to fight against it and the use of it made Madison feel bad about what she was doing, the drug seemed to have a guilt trip affect on her, which was the opposite she had come to observe from Jesse. With her acknowledgement of the affect she continually got" Jesse increasingly tried convincing her it was fine, that no one noticed. Madison wanted to stop, but when he didn't get his way with her Jesse stayed out all night. Therefore, to keep him home she gave him money for what he wanted, most times he never came back. That was fine by Mattie; however, his cheating was constantly on her mind as she struggled to find some since of direction in her life. Madison recognized it was not helping to hold on to that pain; it was tearing up the family. Madison sought help from counselors and family, but the family was too busy to be bothered so strangers helped her to help herself through the destruction she created. What hurt Madison the most out of all this mess was she honestly thought they actually gave a damn about her as a person? The flaw… of always misplacing her emotions, and trust in the wrong people. Mattie's own need to be accepted without expectation was something she yearned to have in her life. To be appreciated by someone was very important and thought this would confirm her true being. That emptiness has been in her heart for years, even as a child. Her nurturing ways is what draws her to folks who seemed to be in crisis. The man who has been in, and out of her life came with plenty of baggage. Madison never dealt with the hand she was given always finding away to make it fit her views no matter how good or bad it was, and because of the false delusions she carried around about people, they latched on to that all too willing to see past others flaws, even when they were working against her. Her therapist helped make her see this about herself' the fact that she too… was looking to be acknowledged" which told her she had some serious issues of her own to work out. Making friends by taking on the problems of others wasn't a good idea, but it was something she'd done for a long time. Did it take a mental breakdown to, make her see what she has done to herself with all that silliness? The realization made her feel like a complete fool putting herself out there to be used that way. It hurt her heart deeply to admit aloud in front of Jonathon, that those people in her life were not the people she viewed them to be, they were manipulative, and conniving bastards who preyed upon her kindness. Jonathan waited for her response to the revelation of not being needed for more than a shoulder to cry on. As he passes Madison a tissue to wipe away her tears, wondering what he now thinks of her for being so stupid. How sad…" she states to him, she tried to be the kind of person people wanted to be around; someone who is trusting and supportive and carries the values respect and dignity she had grown to believe in. Contrary to what she knew to be a way of life" she finally figured out there was little respect for people like her who spoke of trust and honesty. "Shit, society had no room for a sympathetic pushover like Madison who feels gratified in the appreciation of sacrifice. Today she has learned; at least in her generation that most folks have come to have no respect for the common values of truth, friendship, and honor… further believing that saying, thank you" is a sign of weakness. This revelation didn't make her feel any better about the situation. Although, it would have been nice to have someone in her corner supporting her .she disappointingly stands alone to deal with her problems. For a long time Mattie refused to see the world for what it is'… until now. A hard globe of life that is full of destinations, and surprising outcomes depending on what your path is. Unprepared is what she was. Growing up; to be an adult consisted of more than being a mom, having an apartment and working. The whole aspect of living is to live. As children you play' the girls, played house' "here is the mother and the father you have a baby' and a home this is how she thought it to be: there were no examples of struggles' defiance, and destruction in playing house. Madison did fine she felt for someone coming from a broken home. Seeing the world for what it is a learned experience. Life is about challenges trials and failures' something she didn't know anything about, she just some young inexperienced girl out in the world playing adult. By coming fact to face with her demons…she wa forced to acknowledge falseness, reality, and denials she perpetrated upon self" this took a lot out of her emotionally. This is what happens to people who choose to see the world through rose colored lenses as she had… that let others take advantage of her kindness" By never seeing their true motives, and the reasons she chose to ignore. With that came the manipulation one after the other building up a mountain of destructive relationships bound to bring her down. How was she to reconcile from that awakening? There was no way a person could accept knowing her only existence has been through the life of others hardships. Mattie had yet, to know who she was as a person let alone how to move forward. Therefore, it began this continued down turn of tears, and anger for those who betrayed what she thought to be her strongest character trait as a woman. How could people be so heartless as to walk over another helping you? She failed to see it"… What was it that made Madison seek out individuals with such disastrous behaviors like her co-worker and ex-boyfriend? They don't walk around with signs on their back saying. ("Hey pick me… I will suck you dry") no they look just like everyone else you see. Madison wanted all of them to know what they had done to her. She wanted to go after the company for allowing the harassment to take place, but she couldn't prove it was a particular type of harassment hat fail through. Unhappy about the result she ultimately let it go, but the pain of knowing what happened still remains. Realizing she wasn't important enough to those who put her in the position to be attacked it just ate at her heart. How was it that even whole companies can be so unethical and downright shitty' with its' employees do this, if you don't cater to the office politics of kill or be killed" which is what it was for Mattie. The whole "wash my back I'll wash yours" was rampant and she could not get with it. What should have been a sign that something was wrong; was at the end of her first year she got a bonus", but who was thinking about being manipulated, she earned that money. Hell when she started there was already drama taken place with another woman already working in the position she was hired to fill. Another sign ignored. This person was already disgruntled by the fact that Madison was getting her job" now how familiar is that, this woman felt threatened at the fact that she was being replaced by another, and not just another woman, " a black woman at that. She was totally upset by this and Madison could not understand why the woman was angry with her, but now that she thinks about it' that woman was railroaded out of her position too. The company had a circle of road dogs that practiced keeping a revolving door. Employees who played ball and kept quiet about the practices of keeping some of its workers down had nothing to worry about. However, for some like Madison and a few others it was hell to pay. Now ain't that some bullshit practices! Who'd of thought that doing the right thing would cost you your dignity? All the years Mattie put into that company trying to produce quality work, and parts within an environment all concerned could feel comfortable in he never thought it was possible to lose all respect for another human being. Apathetic' is what Madison was after all why would she even think about showing any consideration to any of her superiors, they didn't give damned about her situation, as it was she was constantly being barraged with insults, and innuendos' which were to make her feel as though she should be apologetic about her disconnect from the ol'bunch of cronies. Madison never went out of her way creating havoc just because she could, but she should've made work life a living hell for all of them son of a bitches" that played a part in her destruction. A character trait she did not possess, until she departed the gates of hell' which Is what the company should be called for all the folks lives they underhandedly destroyed for the sake of pure greed" and power tripping. Somehow, "I just don't think the owners of that establishment really know what is happening within the walls of their business. Moreover, if they are and were aware of the practices of abusive tactics on the premises they should be reported and shut down far as Mattie is concerned. Karen a woman lost turned to the likes of two individuals for consoling and support if you want to call it that, and they took that cry for help and used it against her in Mattie's opinion. They played both women against each other for the sake of entertainment without any remorse whatsoever and with the intent of getting both of them out the door. Damn! Observation is truly a beautiful thing" if I do say so myself. All those years "Mattie put up with all the games and psycho babble about how passive aggressive in behavior she was being for not wanting to participate in whatever it was they were dishing out" what the hell is passive aggressive? Mattie had no clue as to what they were speaking of. Anyway, who says "passive aggressive" not Mattie, from what she had come to know of the words; only those who have been treated for some type of mental behavior would have some knowledge to what it means. Madison took on a responsibility that was not hers' and that's alright' she would do it probably for anyone if asked of her… this was her persona 'a kind heart. Someone that wanted to be a friend to Karen in the beginning of that relationship not knowing that there was a hidden agenda to the pairing up of these women. Companies that practice the toleration of abusive behavior on the job regardless of the perpetrators sex should be severely fined for condoning the act' or behavior. With all the observations of the goings on at that job" it never crossed Mattie's mind that she was probably the target. She had gotten to comfortable in her position' the way she strolled around smiling and chatting with the fellow worker's in the building, that didn't sit weill with a few of the company boy's . There were warnings regarding her free spirit travels nonetheless, it was necessary to do the job. Yeah" people talked, but only those who felt they weren't being treated in the same manner as Madison was.

Chapter 5
Are you listening?

"The cries for help"

Madison wasn't up for talking anymore, because it hadn't gotten her anywhere she had given up on getting help on the job. The policy's set forth to protect them as employees seemed to only apply when you are willing to play the game. Madison trusted in those who were in place to help her resolve the matter and they failed to do what they were supposed to in Mattie's case. Madison's tolerance was very low when reasoning with management, Mattie "just as soon curses everyone out, calling them every damned word and mother-fucker…she could get out of her mouth. They purposely let this woman harass her for the sake of productivity. Something she didn't understand about the whole situation. Madison made the decision of leaving the company, sub-consciously trying to figure out what was behind the fighting. This story is hard to explain without sounding crazy, because she thinks and feels that she is the only one who feels there is something wrong in her working environment. For a woman to have tantrums for no reason whatsoever, then went on about her business as if nothing had occurred, ... while proceeding to then carry on a conversation with the person thus called every name in the book. Mattie had such a problem coping with Karen; because this wasn't sometimes... it was all the time. How can someone attack an individual the way she does then walk off for ten-minutes then return to have a conversation with you as if nothing has happened? This is what I had trouble explaining to management. It was not a normal argument, because Madison was hardly a participant. She became a participant after having to defend herself. There was something wrong with this woman; is Mattie crazy, or what? Mattie' had to think about it honestly. Was it in her mind the things Karen said or had done? At first' Madison thought it was jealousy "it could have been the culprit for the aggressive behavior towards her? When she told Karen that she she had been asked to befriend her to keep her from running all over the shop making a fool of herself. Karen was livid about it. She stomped off looking for Paul to see if what Madison had said was true... he didn't admit outright to any participation, but he didn't deny it anything either" he went on to say to Karen that her constant lateness, and behavior was causing problems. That must have been when she made it her business to go after Madison? In fact, Mattie does admit she should have been up-front with the woman. Madison didn't realize Karen had been so hard up for friends' or otherwise. Furthermore, her emotional state of mind was not apparent in the beginning of the working relationship that was somehow kept silent. Madison's intentions were never to hurt Karen; it was to give her an outlet. However, Karen had not asked for help it was assumed she needed it by Vern and Paul. Mattie recognized long ago there was a problem and she came clean about the effort. Karen wanted to make a big deal about it by yelling at her she saying she was just a big liar. Madison never signed on to be a friend sure enough, but the possibility of that relationship had come   and gone due to the way the work relationship started out. Karen became hostile and abrasive very belligerent with Madison on purpose... know why she was angry and figured it should die down in a week or two. She was wrong. Karen continued to insult Mattie's work ethics, with subtle threats of intent. This intense need to defend herself from this woman was stressful as she resorted to maintaining a shield for protection. Unable to explain the tightness in her chest and stomach it made her feel ill. Karen's attitude was more malicious in that she felt' she had the right to impose her harsh opinion upon Madison of not choosing to be a friend. Saying' she had never seen a black women with the authority of telling a white person what to do. This woman had to be lying! It had to be her anger talking? It was all anger talking and truthfully, it wasn't because of Madison it was because she had no since of direction or stability in her life. I think' I gave her the hope of having that in her life, by showed her there was a possibility of being a better person. Instead of embracing the hand, she bit by throwing race in Mattie's face. Madison knows Karen is intentionally trying to make her feel uncomfortable using the race card regarding the job, and being a black female working in a shop full of men. Madison paid no mind to what she was saying at first; she knew that racism was around all the time. Madison did not worry about that there were more pressing issues at hand. Besides, she had a good working relationship with everyone in the shop. I had no time to focus on what others thought of her personally, certainly not for silly matters. She taught herself not to let others opinions about her character affect what she thought of herself. Although deep down she felt self-conscious about her being the only black woman in the shop,... the subject never surfaced and that was fine by her. She felt the lead worker was a little racist' but it was nothing to cry about. The only one having the issue with

Madisons color was Karen it was a convenience. Madison found she was alone in her turmoil accept for a secretary named Ruby. Ruby understood Mattie being angry at what was happening, unable to count the times Mattie' cried on her shoulders about her situation agreeing" something needed to be done. She has also had some confrontations with Karen. The obligation was too much to absorb feeling inundated with frustration, for letting Karen's behaviors take over her thoughts made her feel like a failure at everything. Mattie knows this is part of the reason for her downfall at least most of It. It was so bad that Madison would actually get up in the morning planning a strategy on how to block Karen' from her mind. It really upset her to have to live that way, and for years she put up with her bullshit). Karen came in ready to hassle her on principle. It was so obvious people in the shop were feeling sorry for her) or they were glad they didn't have to work with Karen.

Mattie was injured at work and knew the stress had to play a part in making her less aware of safety on the job. Which was a blessing in disguise, and is what helped save her dignity the little she had left. Still deciding what to use as an excuse was a struggle. However, it was a long time coming; in that there were signs ignored way back when" even before coming to work for that company. I realize I had a problem with my life, and reality before Karen came along. Handling problems was not something I cared to deal with because I had other pressing matters like how I was going to pay the rent, or get to work. I had problems finding a babysitter for the kids at times I had no time for personal shit, it was too much like real- life. Sweeping it under the carpet always worked just fine for Madison until forced to open her eyes to the garbage piled under the rug. Mattie sits staring at the walls surrounding her noticing how dull the color is on the wall realizing she is responsible for what has happened and know other. The pretense of happiness, and failure to handle any problems that came her way was the major cause of the breakdown. I put emphasis in people that I had no business doing. I set myself up for failure without knowing it. Something I have always done even as a kid. Maybe I wanted to be wanted, with no father and a mother I think hated me at times. I just started making more of an acquaintance than I should have. And meeting and working with this woman I guess made me think my life was somehow more stable than it were. The appearance and mannerisms of Madison was for a life she has long dreamed of 'but in fact, was far" far from being. Because, she refused her conscience when it was telling her she had worn out her usefulness in the company that there was nothing she could do to change her outcome. How many slaps in the face was it going to take her to see that they allowed this type of abuse to go on because I didn't fit their needs. It should have been a clue way back when it seemed feasible to escape the back stabbing populous" that had been brewing for years. Madison ignored it. It just never occurred to her; that it was she they wanted out". Madison had plans to retire from that company on her way to building a life for her family she knew it was going to be hard with the pay and all, but never thought she had to fight this woman literally for what she had known as her way of life. Karen was like a chisel breaking down a barrier of protection Madison had built around her maintaining a mindset she had come to rely on for years. While she was losing the resilience, she once held within her to a ruthless, heartless soul. Another clue had passed her by. I failed to see, It pained my heart deeply, because I was forced to behave in way's I had grown past years ago, and wasn't used to acting out irrationally. Mattie felt she was being stabbed from the inside out, and you don't know whether to scream or cry because it hurts so badly. I felt, as if I was in mourning over the death of a woman I once use to be. Madison couldn't breathe it felt, as if a clear plastic bag was being held over her head smothering her to death. The nightmare clouded everything she knew to be her world. None of it was real the friends that safety net she built all made up. The ability to think, to or rationalize the events taking place in her life seemed to blend into a blob of useless confusion. Is Madison crazy for the views she chose to live by are morals long gone are we a nation of taker's and those like myself fools for not conforming to the ways of our counterparts. Was having to give up her job for peace of mind the right choice, or was she giving in to Karen and her personality out of fear she might actually win. She was so ashamed of herself for what she has become she had to get out! Having her soul on display for all to see how shattered she'd become was too much. You would have to be Karen to know that pain as I do now. Madison returned only to turn in her resignation; she had already been off work on family leave prior to quitting, which was to get a grip on what happened feeling this gaping hole in her chest. There was no turning back the boss was walking along side Madison out the door "talking to her about coming back, all the while she is crying about her inner pain. Letting him believe it was something else other than the truth although, this was wrong of her this is how it had to be. Understanding he had no idea of the pain, she was suffering in being there. Vernon was telling her that he would try to help her come back to the same position if possible. "Madison was thinking) as long' as the practice is tolerated it will never be! That let her know further' he had no idea how bad the situation had gotten with Karen. She could not do it! The shear pain of exposing her wounds to those guys who betrayed her was all too much to swallow' the anguish she carried all those years would have killed her. No one could help her now' it was too late. As she walked out the building, she kept the look of durability until getting into her car, and she sat there in a trance. Madison felt that any company that tolerates abusive employees was no place for her. Madison started her car and drove off looking back at what she thought was a place of acceptance and happiness that turned out to be a place of recognition and a truth.

Chapter 6
Inner Battle

Who is in charge? Thoughts of a heart healing

Since leaving that company everything went downhill, Madison was injured and had to leave her job, her love life was in shambles; it couldn't get any worse than that. With all the bad luck thrown at her feet... the only option was to make a change. She had no one to confide in that would be open minded enough to hear her out so putting it on paper helped to start the healing process. Instead of placing, so much enfaces on her invisibility to others; Madison decided to use her own relationship to her advantage. All the hostility she carried she took it, and put it into reinventing herself. However, old habits die-hard when you have been a certain way for many years. That left her with having to forgive those who caused her pain; with a suggestion from Jonathon, he wanted her to consider it a part of her recovery. Madison knew she was going to have to get past the pain in order to move on with her life. The broken heart felt like it had been stomped beyond repair, but her health was worth it. Blaming others would only prolong the pain besides she brought this upon herself, expecting more from people than they had the ability to give. A trait Madison had no control over when she happens to meet someone she cares about, thinking it would be reciprocated, as when her boss failed to stand by her side, or when she fell in love with Jesse, or the fact that she tried to be there for one in need. When that did not happen she took it hard knowing they did not feel for her as she did towards them. It was hard to accept the truth of who she was.

This continued heartbreak was of Madison's own doing. Not having any control over her need to be loved. The pain of not having that shut her down. Mattie, has been so busy defending all the reasons for not opening up about her feelings, that the ability to grab hold to a friendship is no longer there, for fear he wil run them off with her clinginess The anger came when facing the possibility of someone wanting a friendship with her because she knew already what the outcome would be. It had gotten to the point where making friends had become a challenge... even just acknowledging them was unbearable for her. When she sees them, coming Mattie just wants to hurry away, because she doesn't want to acknowledge them...the people; the suspicion is turned up high at the possibility of being approached. As it was when the neighbor knocked on the door asking for her company in a game of cards. This fear of expectation, tends to send a rushing chill through her spine. Stop it! Is what Madison wants to say, but says nothing to the women who had invited her to visit. They are engaging in conversation with Mattie, patiently waiting for a response. Madison staring at the women feeling like a foreigner in her own skin stalls ...trying to tink of an excuse to give to the women.... "isn't that silly. What do you want she asks, feeling foolish at her unease hoping someone will come rescue her from the ambush(we thought you'd like to come down and visit with us, we see you all the time passing by Angie said") .

Which they were quite polite and probably meant well' it was all too much for her to take in. They were seeking friendship from Madison something she wasn't ready to deal with yet. For Madison, having a friendship was too much pressure after the experience with Karen, and Jesse. The relationship's has made Mattie much more suspicious of the motives of all acquaintances. Does she want friends; maybe? How would she accomplish that with so much distrust for women? The ache in her soul left behind a scar believed to be deep as forever from the last encounters...., for it is unsettled, crying most times, because she can't hit, or hurt the ones who brought this pain. That damage done by continued relationships over the past years has made her afraid to associate on a level of one on one. Madison totally locked down at the ability to be accepting of anyone particularly women. Mattie recognizes her own responsibility in the whole ordeal with Karen! It was wrong. The premise was to be a co-worker who showed support ... that part was real. However, the dependency placed upon that support was very overwhelming, and scary. That type of expectation from someone can be very stressful. Today Madison is abitchy woman complaining about everything for no apparent reason other than to vent her frustrations of losing what she felt was a safe haven. This is what has become of her since leaving the job. Madison just wants to hit something or someone out of anger, an anger she held in for years especially towards the man in her life he brought her so much heartache, cheating, and the unwillingness to keep their family together. This betrayal brought nothing, but a hail of storms as she yelled at Jesse for all the pain he caused her as she catches the image of her baby girl sitting in the living room, damn; did she hear anything? Janee, was sitting at the computer playing those doll games as she dose regularly"... now wondering if she heard what she said to her father. What was she doing in the living room? Mattie crying about the fact that she didn't stand-up to the challenges facing her with Jesse and Karen' she couldn't understand it. Who was this person she had become. Why is she so willing to hurt? All she wanted was to make them feel her pain, to see what they had done to her world by allowing their destruction to take place in her world. Spiteful, she has become never having anything positive to say to family members or acquaintances, with an attitude so immature she was criticized as being adversely ridiculous. That shallow behavior has driven just about all who cares away' even her own kids. When your children have a since of unease about their own mother it's saddening No matter how much she promised not to yell" it would just come out. Looking at her with those peering eyes, her oldest son says to her, _ mom why are you so mean to them they are just kids, "in regards to their friends. Madison couldn't handle being around people even children they need to be looked after she wasn't ready for that Madison taught her kids to treat others with kindness and respect' something forgot to do in all herself pity. Defending oneself from an abusive environment for several years has had an astounding affect on Mattie's ability to think first, before responding. She looks back to a calmer Madison... a quieter, soft-spoken personality... that had once been approachable. That Reflection of her former self hurt so much it cut her to the core; to be ripped apart by hate and rage as she were. At one time, there lived a gentle heart inside that wall of anger and bitterness and when she thinks of all the hostility, and mistreatment she tolerated its amazing the breakdown didn't happen a long time ago. Figuring she could survive any situation regardless of the severity being she was always able to fall down, and pick her behind up off the ground from past experiences. It didn't stop her from being who she was "or did it? Thinking about all the paths she has crossed in her unfinished journey, this one has really forced her to acknowledge the person behind the wall. The truth is... she has been afraid of something inside her soul for a long time. This battle with Jesse and Karen opened the doors to a new journey for Madison as she began distancing herself from everyone, because she had shown her ass" to just about anyone she blamed for her failures to maintain her family and lively hood. The family was upset at the way she treated her sister which was quite harshly and disrespectful" Mattie was out of control the verbal abuse was cold, to the core hurtful back then. Knowing the havoc she caused; she stayed away from everyone to get past the hurt eating her alive. All she wanted was to be respected, and appreciated for what she brought forth in other people's lives. Mattie hated that person inside' she had no control over what would happen if she felt threatened. That was a big problem for her, because just being in the presence of people was a trigger. Any type of gesture towards her did it' a flag raisedthat tod her he was in harm's way even if she weren't. However to control the rages emerging inside of her Madison, worked hard to recognize the triggers making her fly into rages. Knowing in her heart there was more to who she was than what was on the surface. Mattie began soul searching from within, because so much was suppressed "by the fear of… if she were to stray from the norm that something pushing at her forced Madison to further take a look at what it was and why. That is when she decided to put her past issues away… and fight that fear of the undiscovered no matter what pain came her way. Deciding to put the heartache on the side has opened her eyes to all the possibilities that lay ahead. Besides she had cried just about all the tears she had" coming to accept what has come to past; only recognizing maybe it was to be. Maybe she was supposed to suffer the downfall, to see what her true calling was to be by realizing as time passed so does the need to be bitter. Leaving the past behind opened the door to another journey, one that seems promising, and quite challenging, ,because she is finally coming into her own.

Madison had yet to know what she has become in her new identity is , but the strong, caring, and selfless being was still there she was only hiding in the shadows of another, because they may feel somehow inadequate about their sorry lives. Madison learned that she can't solve everyone's problems with pep talks, and mediocre advice, That sometimes you have to bow out of those situations and send them on their way.

"*The Reinvention*"

A wise decision made for a new beginning. Starting from scratch' is what she calls it. She had to put her newfound personality into perspective before trying to assert herself into society. Madison needed to work out resolving her anger problems first, so she continued seeing a mental therapist once a week and going to group sessions even though she dredded attending the classes. Telling complete strangers about your misfortunes wasn't her idea of recovery. Mattie did not enjoy telling the group she let others use her as a doormat. Nonetheless, she participated sharing parts of what brought her to being a patient at the facility. As she continued to attend the classes, life at home was tolerable because by the time she arrived all the anger was already vented, and Jesse was nowhere to be found for days at time. Jesse not being there made it much easier to cope with her failures. The kids were a little more relaxed when Mattie was calm and that was only when Jesse was gone. Madison continued to write down her pain on paper as an outlet, instead of yelling, "It seemed to be working for her. The more she wrote the easier it was to talk about what caused her breakdown. The therapist was so kind…with his handling of Mattie's situation he made her feel like she was important as he conferred with her. He had asked several questions about her child hood, and what it was like for her growing up. Madison told him it was good for the most part, until she reached her teen years, and that is when she began to feel like an outsider within her own family. At home was ok, but when you are the darkest child in the bunch things could get very ugly... especially if people remind you that you aren't the pretty one in the family, because you are so much darker than everyone else is. It was definitely hard on Mattie to listen to that all the time realizing they weren't playing around" they were cruel on purpose. Prejudice against dark skinned folks. Racism was prevalent, but she never heard of it in her own race. How ignorant she thought. Grown ass folks who believe that because their skin was a few shades lighter... it made them superior than those of a darker complexion; you couldn't display a more ignorant behavior if you tried. As a child Madison would here things, and sees some of the goings on within her family and it was amazing for the most part, because we always portrayed this quaint forth-righteous family, and was far from being. The point is "they lived a life of pretense that's all there ever was. Madison learned to pretend from the best, even today," her family will never admit to being dysfunctional" all is good in the land of make-believe. Mattie' is working hard to break that cycle of denial; it has destroyed her view of family, communication, and trust. Instead of giving up Madison decided to really find out who she was, and why the man that her family said denied her for all those years, didn't want her... she figured this would help her move forward in herself discovery. The comfort came when however, when she realized she had survived the crisis. It was very emotional knowing she had it inside all the time waiting to be released. The job, the woman, it all had a significant part in her opening up to the world. If not all those events had transpired she would still be living in denial repeating the same mistakes repeatedly. Real life is so much better than pretending when she actually gets to enjoy her new personality. Expression of one's views is glorious. Knowing the truth of what is… makes her heart smile boldly knowing that there was an agenda in place after following the challenges she had gone through. Thinking maybe god wanted her to live a life of hardship, and heartache within the life of others forcing Mattie to wake up, and see life for what it is; not what she wanted it to be.

Madison realized the breakdown was for a reason, and that she had to go through those trials to find out what it is she is supposed to be doing on this earth. Something she was already doing' but not quite the way she was supposed to. The search of what and why began at home for her asking those questions of self… as well as her mother. Madison wanted to know did she hate her when their father left and if not why was she so angry all the time? Her mother eluded the question by saying that her reason for the anger was due to their father and outsiders interfering in their marriage and she was not angry at the abandonment. Madison believes in all her heart' she was very bitter and angry at being abandoned; leaving the kids to take the brunt of her pain. Now much wiser she fully empathizes with her mother's pain. Stupid is what you are when you fail to see things for what it is, as Madison had done for years. This acceptance of responsibility puts her at a different place when making decisions about her life. Madison decided to leave Jesse for good, this is a big part of her downfall' choosing to let go of what could have been, and live with what is; will be a challenge saying it and acting upon it are two different things. Jesse has been difficult for her, he refuses to see Mattie for who she is today, it doesn't matter what she wants far as he is concerned' the thought of losing what he has known to be his life, family and reason for living will not be happening' … as long as he has a breath in his body. Having to face a reality of Madison wanting a better life without him is unbelievable for him. He has always had Mattie to fall back on when his hard life knocked him on his butt" he is in denial of what he has done to her, and expects her to regain her feelings for him just like that" as he puts it. None theless, Madison has already moved forward she has a new perspective on life she is almost happy" if you can even call it that. It seems so unreal to her. That life of hers was so destructive, she can hardly believe what she allowed to occur all those years in that relationship with Jesse. Hardly no effort to blame these days, she explains to Jesse, as best she can why it is time to move forward with her life, that they had grown apart... that her view of where she is supposed to be doesn't include him this time. Jesse pleads with Madison to give him a chance, which he is going to change his ways. That he is tired of the streets and want's the same things in life that she wants if she just gives him that last chance. Only Mattie has heard it all before with those broken promises... oh soo many of them, Madison doesn't know where to begin, and this is not his fault alone. A big part of this disaster was of her own doing. You always want the best out of life, as she planned hers out with Jesse" only never to have it realized waiting all those years for him to grow up. How long was she going to wait, Madison waited and waited for Jesse to catch up, and it never happened... until now. Only after waiting over twenty-five years an emotional breakdown and therapy does he want to change. Only after Madison makes the move to leave him, does he take her serious, before she always gave in to his lies of never doing it again, the cheating and lying all the time. Not this time it was final. Mattie reached a new plateau in her life with the help of prayer, and a lot of soul searching she is on her way and nothing was going to change her mind. Jesse is fighting her all the way, even making idle threats if she leaves him. However, the more threats he make... the more she realizes he has no idea of how much Madison has changed, that there are elements at work thank goodness for the awakening, or she would have never been able to see that writing is what she is supposed to be doing. Since putting her feeling to paper she finds expressing herself and the need of others on a simplistic level instead of holding their hand absorbing all the despair that happens in one's life gives her a better perspective when vocalizing her thoughts on a situation "and or describing another's. Moreover, she has become aware of her capabilities as a confidant of others. Many of whom she knows and spends time with respects her opinion whether they agree or not. She respects that of them all because they feel comfortable talking to her about anything. This is what defines her... the ability to give without expectation, and where appreciation is the key is and has always been a motivator for what she does for people. The problem is I getting Jesse to see that their time together has come and gone... going back is not an option for Madison. Planning and making choices to best fit her need as well as the kids is what's important now even though they are now just about grown, all except one of her kids, their daughter who is and always will love her father' knows all too well that her parents lives have never coincided as one. Something they deserved growing up, but never received. Today Mattie is making strides in redefining who and what she wants out of life' and happiness is her all-time goal. A woman who has no idea of what true happiness is or feels like, besides the birth of her children... nothing has ever been able to top that" if there was anything or one who could. Yet, on that note, there is the one problem standing in her way of happiness..., which happens to be Jesse. Madison has not been able to convince him he is better off without her in his life, even knowing the reason for her choice to end the relationship. How do you talk to someone who believes he cannot survive without you in his or her life? There was no way, especially if they are aggressive in tone at the thought of losing you to another. He was feeling thrown away, or left out of the changes taking places in Madison life. A life he helped push her to pursue. Jesse never gave Madison the time of day everyone else was always first. Mattie came in when he was all wasted, and tired from out in the streets… now how can he say that he is ready for a change when he went to jail, from someone else's home, and it wasn't a partner" , and as she knew it would happen "the person gave hime away like clockwork. Yo know how do when they are after a man all is fair in love and war. Madison gave him one ditch effort to confess it all… and he treated her as if she was a fool' making it up as he goes on with his bullsh*t, believing his own lies, no,… he dare not confess" out of fear of being abandoned in his present state. So with that, Madison made her own mind up that she was done, no more tears, no more excuses was she going to listen at this damn fool" tell his concockted stories. Mattie was better than that, and deserved better than that. And so goes the last draw. Madison doing what she enjoys, being with family and friends, friends she hadn't seen in a long time" because of her choice to distance herelf from others in fear of criticism of the life she had been living. Discovering the purpose of her being was a sign that it was time to move forward to the next chapter in her life. What that is or will be… Madison doesn't know yet, she is still carving her way through the journey that is already laid out for her. All she knows is; it's been a great blessing from the lord who saw fit to keep me moving, who must of been looking out for her the whole time she was going through her hardships. She believes with all her heart that he played a big part in her survival because for a minute" the thought of not wanting to be here crossed her mind" only for a second, this is how bad she was five years ago. Madison felt destroyed by hate and rage the thought of that rocked her to the core, and don't think anyone will ever know just how devastated she was to know people thought less of those who believed in the greater good in all. Not just taking advantage of them, but also purposely trying to destroy them for being that. How evil' how evil are you to be so unforgiving of yourself to go after kindness as you do. All there is for her to say is to pray. Pray for your heart to be healed, it will come he is forgiving of all' no-matter the circumstances... he will show you the way all you need to do is listen he is there not in sight... "But in heart. Even when you feel your heart is empty, it's not. This lesson has been very hard and long learned' that keeping others before him is a big mistake, nothing good can come of it. Lesson taught was she loved Jesse so much she forgot how she was introduced, not by coincidence, but by chance, the chance to show she could see beyond the attraction of vanity and lust and failed miserably and paid quite a price over twenty years of missteps and bad decisions. Madison can move on without the worries of others interfering in her life. she has time to get her life in order there are changes occurring every day to keep her family moving in in the right direction, her writing and spending time with her kids is has been a welcome, no yelling, just a good time. Madison didn't miss anything more than spending time with her kids something she has wanted to do for a long time, even when she was working all those hours being home with her kids was her only desire, but that was impossible... bill's had to be paid. Nonetheless, once she had no choice but to be home she still lost precious time on her mental trauma 'it was devastating... it affected her son as well He had developed that same type of fear at the hands of his parents. Madison is saddened by this disease we call anger it grows and is contagious, and only leads to destruction and heartache. When you are unable to express your thoughts and feelings to people you care about, even when you are provoked... that is the sign: right there. He is afraid to express himself' unless provoked, then he is very harsh, short, and aggressive' just as Mattie was in her turmoil. Holding in your pain is the worst thing a person can do it is a cycle that has been handed down generation to generation,... which looks like no ending insight. The cycle of abuse is not good for anyone and it starts out as fear. When Madison was afraid to speak her mind she use that fear inside to create chaos, build resentment inside which brought out the rage. Hiding behind rage was the easiest way to hide the pain. In fear, you tend to do what you have to; when protecting yourself. That said' he is slowly coming out of his shell since Mattie has given him the avenue of talking with her about the reasons for his closing up when he is approached with some of the most simplistic round of questions. People like him and Madison' they aren't slow, or stupid ... none of those answers are truth' what they are in her eye's is observers' answering the questions in mind, fearing if spoken aloud they are visualized; seen or would become a focal point of knowing" which creates the fear 'even if you aren't right. A character trait Madison has never felt comfortable in... in any situation. She doesn't know why it happens; she only knows that it does. Surely there are folks exactly like the two of them, who carries a fear of speaking up' based on what might happen to them if they should. Madison unintentionally' created that fear within her child at a very young age. She saw that fear in his eyes; it was of her. It was a sad moment for her because of what she had done to him. In addition, he had no clue as to what she had been referring to as a little boy in kindergarten. However, today he totally understands what happened, and he tell's her why he cannot express himself to others, like everyone else does. He gets up-set about it always after the fact... he knows the answers; yet' holds it in. How familiar to Mattie is this story. More like reliving it through her child. This reason alone is forcing Mattie to change the way her family communicates with each other... the aggressive tone, and language is ending if she has anything to do with it. If it takes writing to get this out to others who find that they are in serious harm's way then she will write, Write until it is quite known that any type manipulation is a form of abuse for self-serving purposes. Yes,' there are all sorts of manipulation tactics' but what Madison is talking about is the need to control another's emotional thoughts, to take away the ability to see clearly their true intentions… an agenda, of sorts. This goes back to the job. The manipulation of two people forced to go after each other for their personal entertainment… a deceitful practice that destroyed someone who used to be anything, but ruthless. Madison has nothing, but pity for those who took part in that mess. To all of you out there men, women, friends, and everyone not mentioned. There is never a reason to feel isolated' just because you don't have a voice the voice is in your heart" it keeps you alive, and as long as it speaks to you… the words are bountiful. Tell the world of your pain and see how much free'er you will be. There is nothing like expression to finally say what is on your mind" is truly a blessing in itself… it don't matter where you are, or who you are with if it needs to be said, say it! Madison isn't talking about disrespect,… she is speaking about faith' having faith in what is real, and true. If you speak the truth "there is nothing that can hurt you' except the denial of what is. Madison has always been silent about the things she saw, and it wasn't her place to talk about it… this is what she used to think; those days are over. Madison has plans to confront a part of her family with the truth of what they aloud to happen in their own family this is going to come out whether they like it or not: thus not a witch hunt…" but a means to an end, Mattie would like to have her whole family together again. The division is massive, uncalled for" about unresolved issues, no one want's to talk about. In the mean time, she will continue to put her views to paper reaching as many readers as she can stressing the point that anyone can hurt another, but not anyone can walk away. To go the other way says you have character' not that you are cowards'…like most who knows no better. Mattie to had to relearn how to back away that confrontation is not the way to solve problems. That's funny; not really, because she learned to turn the cheek at a very young age" that just, because you are insulted or treated badly, you don't return the favor... tell them you understand, but disagree. This is what most folks call the cowardly way to handle aggressive situations' such as the one she dealt with, with Karen. She also thought Mattie was a coward. That is fine today "but it was Madison walking away from the whole episode that truly saved her soul. Having the courage to leave a job she loved for the sake of another's safety, was a challenge in itself, after all she was the one who was about to commit the atrocity upon another. Only fate had intervened if you call getting injured fate... for her it helped closed the door on all the chaos in her life. Starting with accepting her part in what happened, only then would she is able to bring closure to that chapter. A journey that's been a learning process of of patients, time, and adaptability of course. We meet all types of people in our lives and you can never be too cautious of who you decide to let in... they might surprise you with a side of themselves you are unable to control and that would be unfortunate. People always asked her how come she never put her hands on the woman, after all she had done Mattie always responded like this, why should she give her the opportunity to have her arrested for assault then she would most definitely look like the bad guy. Madison didn't dare act on her aggressions, oh but how she wanted too. Today though... if she saw the woman Mattie would probably hug her, hug her tight, and whisper quietly in her ear saying " I forgive you' and it's not your fault" then apologize for playing a part in that whole set-up. Madison calls this a part of moving forward. Holding on to anger is poisonous it eats away at your inside causing you to make a fool of yourself, because you're not in your right frame of mind when something sets you off. Believe me there are triggers all around pushing at you, eating at you... feeding all that old garbage you're so bent on holding on too for all intents and purposes of lashing out. When Mattie decided to let it go' she felt a weight lifted off her shoulders. Her writing was beginning to make a since, instead of all that garble she had written down. At the start of her jotting down all her pain she was all over the place with it, nothing really made since to tell the truth. Yet' it all had to do with her pain. Slowly the days passed and she started to unscramble the puzzle of her heartache one line at a time. The more she understood of her path a place in her began to heal it was like watching a new leaf on a tree sprouting for the first time and Mattie would watch it as she did herself becoming anew each day. It is how she felt at times. Like a brand new leaf, Madison began springing up from beneath all that dirt that had been covering her identity. That's when she realized this inner strength was coming from elsewhere' knowing it wasn't just her alone… no he had to be listening to her heart that cry for help,.. It could only be from him' she was not sure about though. Mattie was never one to attend church, but in her heart she always believed he was there watching, wondering why she was so elusive to his warnings. Why didn't she listen earlier to the signs put in place and the only thing she could do is keep trying' trying to hold on to what she believed to be her life. What Madison finally figured out is that she isn't making the call's' they had already been made before she came into the world. It was all up to her to find the way to her true purpose in life. Having an idea of what it is she is supposed to be doing' still confuses her only because it is all she does practically; take care of others……. listen to those who need a shoulder to lean on, and carries the burden of some of these folks…. This calling' is what brought her to today' how can this be? Giving of self is a hard thing to do he knows this whole-heartedly' already doing it so many times' unselfishly to many that sought her out. For this to be her calling in life' is amazing… swearing never to give herself to another ever again the cost is detrimental when you think about what is could bring by opening yourself up to outsiders as she did in the past. What would be different about that path, what? To answer those questions would only open up all the wounds she is trying to heal. No person should have to feel that hurt... it is so wrong. The lesson hard,... has she yet, to learn from the mistakes of the past or is there more to this lesson she tires from. The point is there was a leson learned, and she is not going back to a past of hardship, heartache, and no trust. Madison has been able to find happiness in talking with friends outside of her circle' which helped her to shed some light on her need to hold on to what if's; All whick have been let downs. This search for answers has taken her miles away to finally meeting that one person that was willing to listen, no questions asked, and most of all no judgmental remarks' that weren't called for. He just made himself available to her. This person has come to be one of her most supportive associates today" and she finds herself very much attracted to him. This man doesn't really realize how much of a godsend he has been in her life. Mattie thought her search for true happiness was just dreams. This man has stolen her heart' how could this be? One phone call was all it took and she knew he was the one. That call has changed her forever, and most of all she has rediscovered her true being, the person she was before the breakdown has returned only much wiser and less gullible these days. This is what faith has brought her, in the long search for self-recognition. To think; she thought what she wanted was in a man who almost never ever gave her the time of day unless he was getting something out of it: How sick was that. All her dreams seems to be coming true, but Mattie can't afford to let it sidetrack her from the reality that she still has a problem in her life she yet has to resolve. Jesse needs to let go of a past that no longer exist at his own doing. He is ultimately responsible for this outcome. His lack of respect shown towards the long drawn out relationship, which was one-sided the whole time they were together, never taking on any the hard work it always takes to maintain the relationship, where Madison continued to have hope for something to happen, but it never did. Now that she has finally accepted that he will never be faithful. When you have allowed a person to walk all over you for years; it is bound to catch up with and fortunately she reached her breaking point, the tears had dried up the anger was barely there she couldn't even crack a frown at hearing his little friends message on the phone' she sat there thinking what's the point. Done! Is what she said aloud to herself? Life is too... darn short to let the rest of it past her by. Deciding to pick-up the pace in her new found hobby she adds chapter after chapter of stages gone through. Moving forward in trying to get her personal journey of mental trauma on record for others to view and analyze for whatever reason they feel it would benefit their need, why keep it a secret that she was a fool: Madison is sure that there have been many a couple to have gone through some of the worst relationships today. A many a day she thought about getting out and running for cover, but something always came over her sidetracking the idea of leaving. Popping up the questions who is going to want to raise another man's child let alone two children; Madison wasn't really looking for a man in particularly to run to... she was in search of a bright light one that would lighten her load. The urge to let go of all the worries she carried around for others was dragging her down, nothing seem to ever come close to what she sought. When it came to Karen or Jesse, they were like her adult children always in need of something of her. Frankly she doesn't understand how she became so unidentified that her existence became null' to the others cry for help when Mattie needed someone herself. And yet' again it was her being, this is why she existed so long in her manipulative world of users and unappreciative abusers of kindness. Strong has she become to withstand a breakdown? Madison's resilience to pull through hardship amazes ... she asks why? Why and how is she coming through this still sane; sometimes thinking is he watching her; could it be that he has mercy for her in her time of sorrow, and loneliness. Certainly its not, because shes a big attendee of the church; even though she should be seeing he has come to her rescue on many occasions for various pitfalls of circumstances. Madison's belief in; and of him is overwhelming as she speaks to him regarding her bad choices, and the reasons she believe to have made them. Her main thought however, is when does the selflessness end, that need to put herself out there for others knowing how it has turned out in experiences of earlier times. Dealing with her past associates taught her that it doesn't matter what your intentions are towards others if they need help only offer suggestions, or find someone who can help. Madison has come to appreciate who she has become over the last six years. A woman who often speaks her mind, and doesn't let nothing much intimidate her even if it means hurting another's feelings to get her point across it is only due to the awakening of a sheltered soul' that has found her voice. Yes: there is no other explanation for it; of how she has come into her own remembering feeling ridiculed for being naïve about her choice of tolerating all the problems that came into her life. How weak of them to say this, what makes another so much better than she; because they know how to run... run away from the trials that face all sooner or later. To listen at most women, they would run in a heartbeat if they had to deal with a man like Madison had years ago... what is it they say" better you than me? Please! Those of you who do run I sympathize; however, for those of you with the courage to run, tell me what is it like for you? Does it make you feel stronger, or somehow empowered that at the sign of conflict you jump ship? This is not how it has been for Madison' nothing close to it. Trying to leave a bad relationship scars you in one way or another, for her it is trust in people not the relationship itself. Its believing in when things in life bring hardship you have that lifeline of family, friends, and maybe common since that carries you through the darkness you face day to day; nothing hurts more than knowing you need to get out' but continually fights to save a relationship that is not! Support is what lacked for her, yes, no one was interested knowing she had threatened to leave several times before. You hear it often enough, they don't hear you...like Madison had repeatedly done in the past. Who'd of ever thought she had it in her to walk away'...she didn't you can believe that. A prisoner is what comes to mind for her that is what you don't see appearances are quite deceiving as you may know by now that girl could hide a mountain behind that smile of hers and she did. That mountain carried such pain for her... denial was the only way to survive what laid underneath. Madison could put on a façade no other saw, she was good at it; being she was seen as one who had her life under control..., a face she hid behind for years. Everyone had known her personal life was a joke" but it was how she handled it that gave others no reason to concern themselves about Mattie. Life goes on why let the fact that she had a cheating, lying man in her life stop her from taking care of business. Madison refused to let that bring her down; she didn't want to be defined by his personal dilemmas. His behavior gave her the energy to keep going, she didn't see her pain as a sign to get out... why she wasn't going to let someone else have what she thought was a goldmine" what? Hell no! Only he wasn't anything close to what she perceived him to be when she finally fell to the mountain on her back. Jesse was not her soul mate; no far from it. Ideology" is a son of gun when you want what you want. Blinding to the view in her eyes he knew what to do to take the focus off his weaknesses. She saw in him everything she wanted in a man, truth, honesty... the ability to make things happen, and a drive I have yet to see in any man she has ever met. Madison expected nothing more of Jesse, except for him to meet her halfway on what she had contributed to a one-sided relationship. Hardly' the relationship was doomed from the beginning, because she had goals and dreams known to him at the time, but it didn't matter he was not ready for the responsibility she expected him take on, he was to focused on what was outside of the relationship he couldn't tell if she was coming or going. That is why she finally gave up on a dream to nowhere with a man who seemingly showed no interest in their future together. Surprisingly; he now pretends to have all best intrest at heart' now that her time seems to be elsewhere, other than him. The man is just out of control frantic about her leaving him' he constantly apologizes for all the pain he caused her all those years. Jesse is so emotional in his plea' for Madison not to leave him, she hesitates on her answer to him... feeling a little saddened by his efforts of holding on to the past. Madison certainly loves the man, but it doesn't erase what he put her through; yes she thinks about forgiving and letting him come back; just for a second. That second is jolting' there is no way she can go back to a life of sadness, it is too much to forget. Moving forward is her only focus whether she has someone in her life or not? The future is all she has to look forward too...no one will interfere with that plan. Writing and thinking about all the possibilities are endless at this poin... how can she think of anyone at this point in her life' with a child about to finish school' and on the way to college freedom is all she can think about, after all the battles fought in her search for happiness. Still she owes this effort to another for giving her the courage to make that choice. Madison is feeling quite emotional about some of the decisions and if they were hurried in that, she was too vulnerable to see her choice clearly when deciding to see another, maybe he won't want to be with her, does he love her... as she loves him? A question that rests in the back of her mind of course hopefully she will learn the answer to this and many of her thoughts soon enough. Keeping focus on her new beginning has been up, and down feeling extremely happy about where she is headed, but still saddened at the course she's had to take to ensure her ability to continue with her life. Fearing Jesse will ultimately interfere with her leaving him. He seems to believe that Mattie is taking his life away as he had known it to be refusing to see the whole picture and the reason Madison has finally decided to walk away. A man who is stuck in a past where he tends to see a young family he wants to raise and be that father figure too... allowed growing away from him. Now grown seeks nothing of him, because he wasn't available to them when they needed him. It hurts Madion to listen to his desperate cry for another chance to start fresh. She was unable to look at his face with his tears running down his cheek.... it's as if he see's life in the past, and he can just play fatherhood without acknowledging the present. That is possible, only he needs to see them as they are today... full grown adults, not children... he has his youngest daughter only she has grown up" not a baby mind you; they always need their fathers no matter the age. Madison continued talking with Jesse every week or so to get him to see she had to move on with her life' without him in it. Telling him he isn't responsible for her decision it was and is all of her own doing, Jesse needed to look inside his heart for the answers and only he can do this. Mattie has asked Jesse to seek out his answers' in the bible; to let it be. His kids are not going anywhere he is and always will be their father. The kids love him, but they are disappointed in him as a parent. He should have recognized they weren't going to be babies forever, they grow up. At certain ages in a child's life they see and hear the arguments, they eventually put things together from there they draw a conclusions' about their parents. Madison has never hidden the truth about their father for fear an outsider could say something to them about him. However, Jesse didn't appreciate them knowing about his problems he figured they wasn't smart enough to know that he had problems. Madison knew better, she had to prepare them for the inevitable; having someone hurt her kids out of spite was out of the question. You can't hide something like this forever, kids are inquisitive they ask questions "where's daddy going? Mattie could only give the same answer for so long, until they start to see you are not telling the truth about it, he was gone two to three days out of the week. All she could do was keep going keeping them focused on other things more important like education, their grades things of that nature after while they stopped asking, it wasn't easy to raise three kids alone, but sometimes you have to put what felt like a chore aside and look at it as a challenge that is what she did. Mattie was tired of feeling like she was encapable of doing for herself, know that was not who she was as a woman. Raised with seven other siblings, she wasn't close to being helpless at all. This is where the strength came from....after all she took care of her own siblings as a child and this was no way as challenging because they were hers she had, had more experience with kids then maybe the whole neighborhood she'd come from. So being tested is nothing new for Madison, she just wanted to be able to accomplish something in life without all the challenges that seeded to be thrown her way. To observe her struggle from childhood to adult, you have to wonder sometimes how she kept it together, but then look at the long line of women before her who had even worse than she did. Her triumph however, came at a small cost: A price she wishes she hadn't had to pay to get where she is now. A son traumatized by the fights that took place long ago; you cannot get that back all you can do is support, and answer the questions of why, Why didn't you pay attention to what was happening around you, was the last word so important you couldn't take the time to put him to bed. A question she will always have in the back of her mind, every time he hesitates to answer a question. This is what it was like for Madison for over fifteen years and counting at work and home there was always something wearing on her mind. To write about it... is a progress in action; moving on to a new chapter, she is wiser and much stronger for walking a road well traveled. Madison picks up from where she left off, by getting rid of all the relevant reminders of that pain she endured all those years. She thinks not.... those memories are what keeps her grounded, never forgetting will help to lessen the next page of what she hopes to be her chosen chapter in the making, as a published writer, married maybe to her desired dreams of what a real man is supposed to be something she has wanted practically half her life. The real woman inside Madison has arose from the depth of a hidden crevasse in her heart, where she had slid into hiding all those years to protect what was left of her soul from a hard fought battle. Madison was quite emotional to feel alive inside from a deep sleep she would never arise from, only to realize she was there all the time waiting to be set free from all that baggage she was holding on to. Her tears ran down her face of the realization of what was happening to her at that moment took her by surprise; to come alive in heart that way, she knew he was doing that for her even now to speak of it brings tears to her eyes to be in her own skin. That heart of kindness has returned healed of its wounds and beating so strong with anticipation of what's to come, she thanks the lord with all the heart he has given her to share with the world. That is the point of the story of her trials, letting others see life for what it is... from inside the soul, not just the outside view. There is and has always been a side to any hardship, heartache, and failures suffered in life. To open up about the breakdown of what, who and why it occurred is what healed the soul. Speaking to the mistakes she encountered forced her to see that her logic about how people are supposed to be "showed that she was undeveloped in figuring out the basic behavior of maturity by suppressing her need to let the outside world in... Thinking if she did then her innocence would be lost. That innocence is what Madison prided herself on, not the innocence of experience, but of giving' a selfless trait that made her the person she was, a D.N.A., that was given her by the lord himself, she knows this, and there is no other explanation for what some people call, pushovers, weak, and easily manipulated. A kind heart is what it is, She is maybe one of millions' that where their heart on their sleeves. Madison probably cries more than any woman she has ever known. Moreover, has been there for a many people in need just, because they needed help. She is her grandmothers, grandchild... she never turned away a soul that she could remember, Madison can't say that... but she knows why her grandma is so loved by so many people. Madison as a child was so attached to her Madea' she would cry her eyes out to be with that beautiful woman. She never wanted to be home. So if anyone ever say's you are a pushover, then you know what kind of person lives inside you" trusting, you give, because you want to believe that they are true in heart. The downside to being a caretaker, nurturer is you don't learn to say no until you have given all you have of yourself then ending up bitter, lost and angry at the world for not making better judgments in the decisions' to give. A warning if you are Mattie, in the making... just stop and look at what you are creating in your need to solve the problems of others. To enable another is to harm their desire to take an initiative of themselves. It is detrimental to the person receiving the hand up or out depending on the mental state of said persons. I have found that long term enabling brings a bad outcome for them, and the giver, they feel rejected and thrown a side. Leaving only resentment, and anger at being left to step up to the plate. Madison can't say enough about how she allowed her situation to continue the way it had If she could do it over there would be some major changes in the way she lead her life. Nevertheless, that is the past... moving forward is what's important to her now, feeling extremely confident in what the future has to offer. How can she not be with the happiness she has found in her search for completion? Mattie overwhelmed by the opportunity to start fresh with another while Jesse refuses to let it be. He is so apologetic for all the hurt and pain he caused Madison during their time together that he consistently asks for another chance to make the relationship work. Mattie listens to his pleas and contemplates his words true meaning. Madison listens to his tears of sorrow as he spouts off at the thought of losing her to another, but all she can think of is all the women he chose over her, refusing to see her heartbreak every time he walked out that door. Jesse never came back until he needed to sleep his fun filled escapades of lust and drug fumed excitement away by climbing into bed next to her as if it never occurred. This was the disrespect; She put up with this behavior from him she became numb to it all" calling it mid-life crisis to immaturity, the point was he didn't want her obviously, because he had her already. He knew this. Madison felt bad as he poured his little broken heart out to her, and she say's (Do you remember... when I begged you not to go all those nights' you looked at me and said Mattie" I will be back.) that was eons ago. Two years ago, she warned him she was coming to the end of her rope with his disrespectful cheating ass way's. It's sad to see a hardhead get his justice: Madison felt her time had come the shoe is now on the other foot and not of her own doing" this is what makes the freedom so worthwhile in her heart. Although, not a punishment for what he had don't to her: No this is a lesson in not appreciating what you had and treating her as a doormat. To lose the one person you thought would be there for you while you troll up, around with all your hussies, and lonely females jumping at you with the first sign of an empty promise of fun filled passion and hopes of a relationship... where he failed to tell them he is in a relationship of several years with children. All the time he took to break her down, he was building his own long awaited lesson in heartache all on his own. To say she gave him time and opportunity to get his shit in order would be an understatement. The tears were waterfalls for Madison thinking she had cried them all out' however, these weren't tears of sympathy for his pain, no...No, they were of the freedom she finally had come to in her long journey of sadness and sorrows for allowing him to do that to her. So she kindly say's to him ... Jesse, I wish you no pain and would always be a friend to you, but we will never be again and you should talk to the lord about the pain you feel inside. To look inside yourself to find the answers to move you forward in life, then she says goodbye to him as he continued to reach out for another chance. His voice stayed in her head as she hung the phone up. The need to reach out is sometimes overwhelming for her she had done this so often with Jesse, that it brought tears, but Madison had to be vigilant in her quest for freedom... let it go, girl... just let go" she thinks. What will life be like without that burden she used to fill that void in her life with"... is what she thinks about? Who would want to be with a woman such as herself, one who gives herself to someone who treats her that way; these thoughts ran through her head quite often, being she hadn't been with another in years" accept for one' who will stay anonymous. In flight...a suspended state of mind with her spirit which is quite alive with thoughts of another being in her life. Madison seemingly almost hesitates for that quest for fear of rejection... something she can't handle at this time. As she timelessly verbalizes that moment of recognition...of a failed attempt at happiness, only saying it aloud to make the hurt less painful as it lifts her spirit to a new height. Only to dissipate all the wasted matter of the past. Irrelevant "in that it didn't define the outcome of what she has now bloomed into from the cocoon of her physical being. Madison now breathing a sigh of relief at the freedom she now possess; what to do' what to do, is the question. Whatever Madison decides to do... it won't include giving up what makes her the woman she is. That the seeker has to know... before they approach that personal side of her soul; he will be scrutinized, and tested in order to touch her soul in such a manner that he might want to think about his desire to know the woman. Precautions are in place in case things aren't going the way it should be, yet' open enough to allow a mistake or two under the circumstances, realizing no one is perfect. The expectations are truth, there is no getting around it moving forward into the next chapter would be impossible without honesty. Living with lies and pretense are the biggest causes of relationship breakups today, and probably will be as long as it is aloud. Nothing is hidden forever if it is done in dark; it always comes to light". How long do you think you can get away with deceits, when the truth is written on your face? Madison always knew with Jesse, she just let him believe what he wanted she had passed the fighting stages of that circus of a relationship. Since the break-up Madison proudly and freely concerns herself for others well being and needs, never forgetting to take time out for self. The one person she had forgotten about in her disastrous journey. Change is intimidating; reaching for something better than what you had' afraid of what the risks might be stepping out of that circle of ... just settle". Trying to become a writer is hard, especially when using your own tragedy as a topic to begin a new life. The story is not rare" but relevant to abuses in our country. The fact that there are folks who use scare tactics to get what they want from someone is abusive, manipulative and scary. This is how it was for Madison for several years; the fear of violence for trying to leave a bad relationship on top of the constant fighting with a woman who was mentally incapable of controlling her aggressive attacks was hard to manage without losing your mind. Having that fear engraved in your head was difficult to shake no matter how much help or counseling she had. Not all therapy resolves the fear... medication for her only prolonged her need to accept the cause of her breakdown. Working to become a writer has been hard with all the changes she had gone through...it brought many difficulties to her story in the process of change. There was something in the way of her need to confront those reasons for trying to be different from her present state. Blockades; is what they are for those who fear losing her to someone or something else' that barrier of why and what are you trying to do is the questions she hear all the time, that skepticism of her new challenges being thrown at her for trying to pull herself up by her own boot straps. Then comes ridicule you can't be no writer she heard it all, no faith whatsoever in Madison's capabilities to be a book writer. Nevertheless, she was able to leave that dreadful relationship with Jesse, not easily done. As for him, maybe he can make the changes in his life to move on wishing nothing, but success for him. Resentment is not worth the time when starting a new life is so much more fun and exciting when reinventing yourself for the new challenges ahead. Madison Billson, a woman who won't be kept down by others need to drag her down. Life is just too short to allow that to be. Her happiness, with the presence of God"... is the essence of her new awakening and creativity. While feeling much more certain now that she has made changes within her life; a success is possible even for her. There are those who are persistent in intruding into her journey, they come out of the woodwork to cause havoc. Not surprised, but unexpected; especially from the ones she sought help from repeatedly with no success. How thoughtful of them to all of a sudden be concerned about her recent freedoms from their family member, recognizing what's bringing them out of the woodwork: How sickening it is. Madison angers at the sudden interest in her new hobbies, for years they kept their distance not one effort to help her with the situation, yet' they feel the need to pry. Change it makes one restless, or concerned about why it is happening"...They are being forced to acknowledge a responsibility they have avoided for years, a reality they continued to ignore for as long as it was possible. Now that the safety net is gone, they have to accept the reality that Jesse may or may not need them to step up to the plate. With questions of who is keeping you occupied, why are you leaving, me asks Jesse, one with many questions... how interesting that folks are concerned about Mattie's well-being. Madison appreciates any concerned for her well being, if it is genuine. With this in mind, Mattie does listen to others views and takes on her newfound efforts at freedom, but that is... all it is for her... an opinion. Respecting is one thing; taking it to heart is another, learned the hard way. Offending her critics is not the intention, but sometimes she has to... to make her point that no one is going to decide what her path will be no one. Arguing with those closest to her about the decisions she making regarding her destination is not up for discussion. Madison is taking time to look at all the mistakes she's made in the past, trying to foresee the one's that may come in her journey' forcing her to second guess any decision she makes. However, with all her insecurities this need to seek out others' is a part of her own self healing, and yes Madison is going to go through many changes including falling for some who may seem sincere in their concern for her outcome, crying and lashing out for reasons un-called,,..Yet, is the process of moving forward? Madison can't say when she will be completely healed from the past... all she knows is that nothing or no one is going to get in the way of her happiness. Madison fights all the critics of her path to freedom and happiness...

insisting she has no idea of what she is doing, from one who has no idea at all of how to maintain or treat a woman in any relationship. The pursuit of happiness has been a long and hard, Feeling all was lost for staying in that suppressive and manipulative prison she lived in all those years with Jesse. The problem that comes with starting over is staying focused on self; Mattie, never thought of her needs before anyone, what to do? With freedom comes temptations and desires to fulfill that emptiness with someone. Anyone . Writing has helped most definitely, but pouring your feelings on to paper brings all sorts of emotional questions" what is she going to do now, all the time she wasted on others problems has now been resolved at last with her and Jesse splitting-up for good. To think of all she could have been doing in her lifetime' is saddening that it took an emotional breakdown and lots of soul searching to get her here. Loving every bit of it, she cautions her every step at least for the time being remembering the past mistakes of jumping into something to quickly as she did with Jesse, and Karen. Focusing on lately on the future and what lays ahead for her. Madison has always wanted someone who loves her as much or more than she loves them a deep desire that has gone unfulfilled it seems like forever, and not finding it with Jesse continues to leave her feeling empty, yet' Madison always hopeful that it is still possible to find that one person who will surprise her. Madison talks to Jesus, quite often in her time of silence seeking answers of why he chose for her to go the path he set aside for her realizing he does nothing in vein' all she has gone through was and is for a purpose..Maybe dealing with Karen, and her personal pain was to wake her up to witness the entire episode of what closing your eye's can do when refusing to see" Truth, right in her backyard" no one is that blind. However, there she stood allowing herself to be mistreated and abused all for the sake of family was the excuse,... her misplaced feelings and dreams of a life unrealized. Hurt is all she could feel even though it's the best decision she's made today. Madison thinks of all her desperate efforts of holding on to a façade an ideal, and cries uncontrollably finally accepting that he never had it in him to love her the way she needed him. How it hurts to see how foolish she's been to let this go on for so long" how he must have thought stupidity' and he did. Sure now that she has, left he won't admit in his time for one to forgive all his wrong doing... he wouldn't dare say it aloud. Madison still cares for him in her own way, but she will never forget all his wrong. The time to forgive has come and gone. Forgiving him gave her the power to move forward with God's help. She always felt that someone had been there for her she just wasn't sure as he continued to open her eyes to the way of his world. Learning that there is none without him, and every time she thinks about it' surviving all her mistakes, and downfalls she cries feeling his hand on her back unaware of whtat it was, all she knew is she had to keep going no matter the difficulties. Madison was doing what she was meant to be doing' caring for others. Always wondering why she never said no, to people in need made her wonder all the time if she was just too soft to walk away from a challenge. Thinking back Mattie had been there for many a folk who needed help. To be there for another' does it make her gullible? No on the contrary it makes her a nurturer something to be proud of, not all has it inside to be as kind or giving without expectation within them it is a gift, or desired quality inside the person. This trait imbedded in Mattie has been like a target on her back' how could one run from a destiny already engraved for them. Madison had been running from it for a very long time, always looking at it as a chore or something to that affect starting with caring for her younger siblings. How could she know this was her calling? Madison yearned for her father as a girl; yet never appeared to answer the questions a young girl would need answered when trying to get involved with a man. She missed all the father daughter talks that her peers had. Something thought about through the years as she struggled to find who she was supposed to be in this world. That feeling of not belonging does much to the spirit' to feel incomplete. For Madison hiding from life was her way to escape the sadness inside her empty heart. The episodes with Karen, was to shake her out of living in denial' this much she knows, and the life with Jesse... well it was a trial she had to finish to realize it was none there. Love did not exist "it was all one sided on her part... a reality she fought for years thinking with time her dream of being with a man who loved her for the person she is. After all the years of fighting, and arguing the relationship ended terribly with her taking control of her life using extreme measures because he was forcing issues that were dead long ago. Life brings the unexpected' at times the most difficult to deal with. The signs unseen, but felt by her inner conscience was gnawing at her; where you are going girl, what are you doing. Did Madison, have it in her to keep moving, and with this in mind... her heart already had been stolen by another who happened at the perfect time. Madison was seriously thinking about taking Jesse back as she does all the time. At the time of separation she met this perfect stranger who came into her life; he saw her and saw something in her eyes calling for his attention. This man kindly gave his time to her... never once criticizing her for the mistakes made in her life, only stating the obvious. At first, she had reservations of letting this person into her world for many reasons' one being she hadn't been socially adventurous in several years, Moreover, he has been in her corner then on out' and has helped her to get past all the heartache, and stress of feeling guilty for finally stepping up and standing up for herself. However Madison does realize their always an agenda in meeting the opposite sex; however in her case this is one meeting she whole heartedly welcomes into her life. A life she now believes is possible since coming into her own, and accepting what has been put forth for her to explore" how could she have tolerated such a person in her life for all those years. After all the hardships , missteps, and bad decisions there can only be success ahead of her now and Madison intends to take every possible avenue to achieve her goals in life.